THE MIND OF THE MOGUL

THE MIND OF THE MOGUL

Fueling Success & Inner Peace In High Powered Leaders

DR. TOLA T'SARUMI

Bethune Publishing House, Inc.

Contents

Dedication

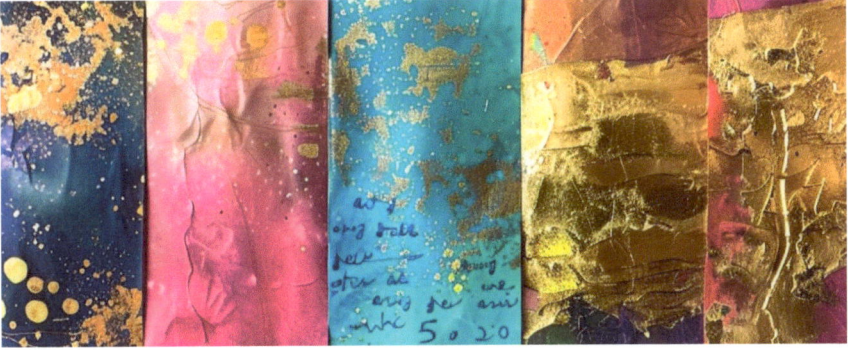

To my parents, who taught me the strength of resilience and the power of unconditional love. To my sisters and brothers, Lola, Bibie, Lanre and Jide, whose unwavering support has been my anchor through turbulent seas. To my husband, Tunde, whose patience and understanding have been my steadfast companions on this journey. And to my children, Tara and Toshe, who inspire me daily to strive for a brighter future.

I extend heartfelt thanks to my mentor, Mrs. Olajumoke Adenowo, whose wisdom and guidance have illuminated my path and enriched my soul. To all those who have supported me in countless ways—Toyin, Ayo, Dr. Shameka, and many others whose names I hold dear—you have been the pillars of my strength and the light in my darkest moments.

Concluding Thoughts:

This book is dedicated to everyone who has struggled with mental health challenges, whether personally or through the experiences of loved ones. It is a testament to the resilience of the human spirit and a tribute to the courage it takes to confront and overcome adversity. May these pages offer solace, understanding, and practical guidance to those navigating the complexities of mental health. Together, let us continue to foster compassion, break down stigmas, and build a community where everyone feels supported and valued.

Forword by Trevor Otts

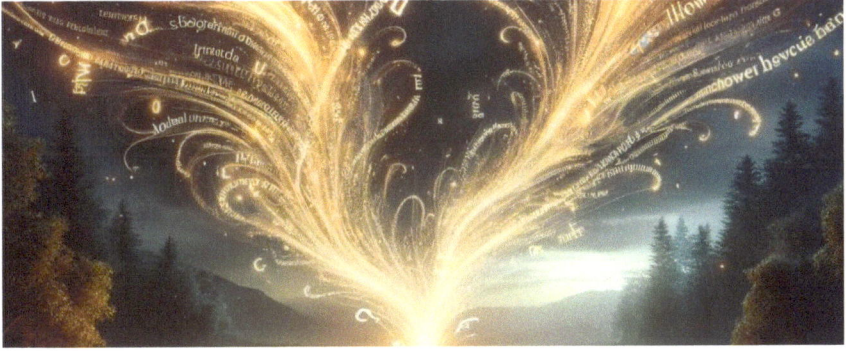

Greetings Dr. Tola:

It is impossible for anything that you finish to return unto you void.
But everything that you leave unfinished in relationship to your purpose
will return unto you as a deficit.
If you finish small things well, you'll do great things.
The end result of finishing is abundance

Congratulations Dr. Tola! Your Return On Finish (ROF) is priceless!

Diving into the heart of what it means to truly succeed, "The Mind of the Mogul" stands as a testament to the unseen battles fought by those we often see standing at the pinnacle of achievement. As someone deeply immersed in the art and science of lifting others to their highest potential, I find this book to be a beacon of light for the high achievers who navigate the tumultuous seas of success, often at the cost of their inner peace.

This narrative is a heartfelt call to action, urging us to redefine what success means in a modern world that's quick to applaud the external and overlook the internal. It's an invitation to embark on a journey of self-discovery and personal fulfillment that resonates deeply with the mission we uphold at BlackCEO.

Dr. Omotola T'Sarumi doesn't just write; she converses with the soul of the reader, guiding you through the mazes of mental health with the grace of a seasoned navigator. This book is not just a read; it's an experience, meticulously designed to transform you from the inside out. It challenges the conventional metrics of success, pushing you to find harmony between your professional achievements and your quest for inner peace.

To the leaders, the CEOs, the trailblazers who've mastered the external world, yet yearn for fulfillment beyond accolades and achievements, this book is your anchor. It teaches that inner peace isn't the antithesis of success but its most reliable companion. In its pages, you'll discover that true leadership is about more than guiding others; it's about navigating your own path with wisdom and compassion.

The journey to self-mastery is complex, filled with challenges and insights that demand vulnerability, resilience, and authenticity. These pages serve as a roadmap, empowering you to confront and overcome the stigma of mental health, manage the intricacies of stress and addiction, and ultimately, celebrate your life amidst your professional success.

In a world that often glorifies the hustle at the expense of well-being, "The Mind Of The Mogul" rewrites the narrative. It's a clarion call to those who dare to lead not just with their minds but with their hearts. It's for those who seek to leave a legacy that transcends professional success, one that encompasses personal growth, fulfillment, and, most importantly, happiness.

So, to my fellow moguls in the making, let this book be the compass that guides you to the uncharted territories of your soul. Let it light up the paths less traveled, the ones that lead to true fulfillment and peace. Embrace this journey with an open heart, and let the transformation unfold

Black CEO For Life!
Trevor Otts,
Founder

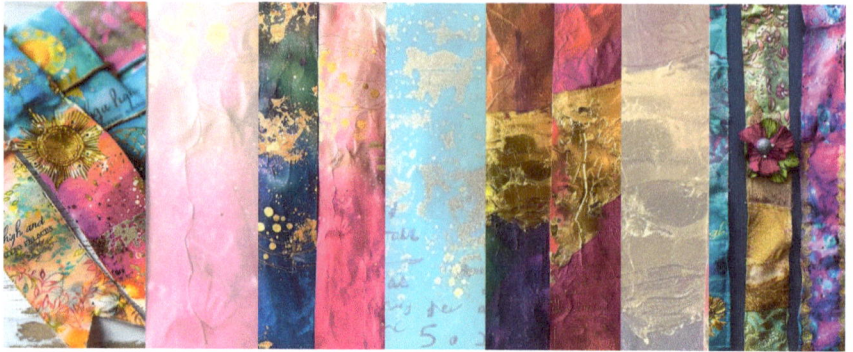

I

⁄⊗⊗⊗

From Stigma to Courage: Shattering Mental Health Barriers and Embracing Your Inner Strength

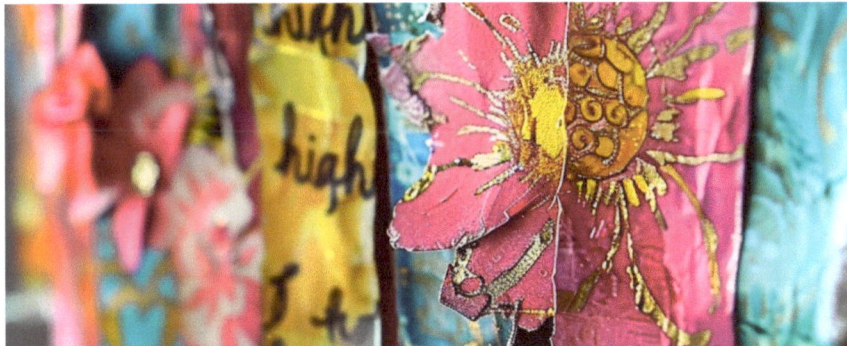

"In an authentic voice, challenge stigma with courage; embracing vulnerability fondles inner strength, and ushers in compassionate conversations."

In the heart of bustling metropolises, in glittering corporate towers, operating rooms, and boardrooms, they stand - stalwarts of accomplishment and emblems of professional success. They are leaders, visionaries, guardians of multi-billion-dollar corporations, and trailblazers in fields as varied as medicine to technology. Their lives appear to glow under the gleam of prosperity, their achievements a testament to their mental acuity and relentless drive.

However, beneath the surface of this visible success, a battle rages. It's a battle fought in the shadowy recesses of the mind, fraught with stress, anxiety, depression, and an array of mental health issues that are as real as they are invisible. Among these silent struggles, one of the most devastating and often overlooked is the risk of suicide.

Suicide claims the lives of thousands in the United States alone yearly. It's the third leading cause of death for children between ages 10 and 14 and the second leading cause of death for people between the ages of 15 and 34. Tragically, these statistics don't improve for physicians and other high-achieving professionals. In the U.S. alone, an estimated 1 physician dies every day from suicide, with a yearly total about equivalent to an entire medical school.

As a society, we applaud their triumphs and laude their careers, but we often ignore the stark reality of their mental health battles, relegating their struggles to hushed conversations. However, the time has come to shift this paradigm. The time has come to muster the courage to bring these battles out of the shadows and into the limelight, to challenge the stigma associated with mental health, and to foster a climate where it's okay to admit that even the strongest among us need help.

My own family has not been immune to this silent epidemic. Let me share with you the story of my uncle, a tale that has profoundly shaped my understanding of mental health and the devastating impact of suicide.

My uncle was a brilliant physician who had studied abroad. Like many families growing up in Africa, his parents saw his acceptance into a prestigious medical school as the pinnacle of success. He completed his course and secured a residency in Primary Care in a foreign land, seemingly living the dream.

From the outside, his life appeared picture-perfect. He was married, had a child, and was building a successful career. But beneath this facade of achievement, a storm was brewing. The isolation of being in a country populated predominantly by Caucasians, far from his immediate family, played a significant role in his struggle.

As the years progressed, subtle changes began to appear. Family members who visited noticed he wasn't as cheerful as before, but they attributed it to the normal stresses of life. Little did they know that these were early warning signs of a deepening depression.

Depression, when severe, significantly increases the risk of suicide. The early warning signs are often subtle but crucial to recognize:

- Persistent sad, anxious, or "empty" mood
- Feelings of hopelessness or pessimism
- Irritability
- Feelings of guilt, worthlessness, or helplessness
- Loss of interest or pleasure in hobbies and activities
- Decreased energy or fatigue
- Moving or talking more slowly
- Feeling restless or having trouble sitting still
- Difficulty concentrating, remembering, or making decisions
- Difficulty sleeping, early-morning awakening, or oversleeping
- Appetite and/or weight changes

• Thoughts of death or suicide, or suicide attempts

This personal tragedy has deeply influenced my career path. As the first physician in the family and a psychiatrist, it has become my passion and goal to raise awareness about physician suicide and the unique stressors that come with high-pressure professions.

The loss of my uncle underscores the critical importance of mental health awareness and suicide prevention, especially among high-achieving professionals. It highlights the need for open conversations about mental health in environments where it is often stigmatized or ignored.

Bound by the invisible chains of mental health issues, even the most successful individuals yearn for a life that goes beyond mere survival - a life that is not merely tolerated but celebrated. It's a journey from suffering in stoic silence to courageously embracing one's vulnerability and inner strength. It's a journey where the authenticity of being human, with all its attendant struggles, gains precedence over the illusion of unassailable perfection.

The task may appear daunting, even insurmountable. Confronting the hidden struggles, breaking free from societal conventions, and acknowledging personal battles require immense courage and resolve. However, this chapter and the subsequent journey promise that it is possible to traverse this path, garnering strength with each step taken.

This chapter is your invitation to this transformative journey. Embracing the principle of courage over stigma, we will delve into the covert struggles faced by high achievers. We will shatter the barriers of stigma, encourage brave, candid dialogues, and most importantly, acknowledge and celebrate the immense inner strength that resides in each one of us.

Prepare to be inspired by stories of resilience, moved by tales of struggles, and emboldened by narratives of transformation. Expect to find tools and strategies that help you navigate your mental health journey, foster resilience, conquer fear, and reclaim your life.

This chapter is not just about raising awareness; it's about wielding that awareness as a tool for transformation. It's about owning your story, honoring your individuality, and discovering the incredible power that lies in being authentic.

As we embark on this transformative journey, let's remember, "In an authentic voice, challenge stigma with courage; embracing vulnerability fondles inner strength, and ushers in compassionate conversations."

Together, let's shatter the silence, break the chains, and commence our journey toward a life that is celebrated, not merely tolerated.

Speaking the Unspeakable: The Power of Vulnerability

In our quest to dismantle the illusory ideal of invincible success, let's pause for a moment on an underappreciated part of our humanity; vulnerability. This term often carries a negative connotation, equated with weakness and seen as a detriment to our aspiration to succeed. But in reality, vulnerability is not just inevitable, it's invaluable. It's a currency of courage, a testament to our authenticity, and most importantly, an invitation to connect with each other on a deeper, more meaningful level.

Brené Brown, a renowned empathy scholar, once said, "Vulnerability is the birthplace of love, belonging, joy, courage, empathy, and creativity." By admitting your struggles, you are welcoming other people to be a part of your journey, to understand you, empathize with you, and walk alongside you.

Think about it. Behind the accolades and triumphs that we admire in successful people, there is bound to be a story of struggle unheard, a phase of low ebb unknown, but it is there, ever-present. By speaking about our struggles, we offer this hidden, human aspect of our story a voice, creating a bond of shared understanding and empathy.

Moreover, speaking about our mental health battles can also be profoundly healing. It's akin to opening a pressure valve, allowing your pent-up emotions, insecurities, doubts, and fears to find release. It gives us the space to breathe, reassures us that we are not alone in our battles, and invites others to show empathy.

Imagine you're at the peak of Mount Everest. You've reached the summit, defied the odds, and accomplished what few others could. From this vantage point, the world seems small, and your achievement is monumental. Yet, as you stand there—admiring the panoramic view, breathing in the thin, unforgiving air—the exhilaration begins to wane, and a different reality dawns. The invisible wear and tear, the physical exhaustion, hypoxia, frostbite, the looming threats of avalanches and crevasses—these are the silent, unseen companions of your victory.

The life of a high achiever mirrors this mountaineering metaphor remarkably well. At the zenith of success, standing in the spotlight and basking in applause, these individuals bear silent witness to their own invisible struggles. In their minds unfold scenes that aren't part of the highlight reel.

Mental health issues often remain confined to the hidden shadows of success. The exhilarating rush of signing a new deal, the thrill of orchestrating a successful campaign, or the satisfaction of solving a critical problem can become a smokescreen, concealing the underlying symptoms of stress, anxiety, depression, or addiction.

These high achievers lead a dual life - a life that's publicly acclaimed, but privately stricken with apprehension, self-doubt, and unease. They navigate the treacherous terrains of their minds, much like a mountaineer traversing a perilous glacier, with each step fraught with hidden crevasses and subtle dangers.

They are trapped between unsustainable expectations and the vulnerability of their humanity. The world sees the glowing success, but not the relentless stress that courses through their veins. Society praises their unyielding strength but remains oblivious to the battles they wage within the solitude of their minds.

My uncle's story is a poignant example of this hidden struggle. To the world, he was a successful physician, living the American dream. But beneath that veneer of success, he grappled with isolation, cultural displacement, and the immense pressure to maintain the image of the successful immigrant. His battle with depression was invisible to most, masked by his achievements and the expectations placed upon him.

However, this dual existence is not an inescapable fate. Acknowledging these hidden struggles is the first step towards instigating change. To illuminate these dark crevices, we require the torch of understanding, empathy, and courage.

Understanding creates the foundation for empathy, empathy fosters connection, and connection, in turn, fuels the courage to speak, to raise awareness, and to initiate change. When we take off the masks of artificial perfection, when we open ourselves to the vulnerability of being human, we encourage others to do the same.

Our battles with mental health are not a sign of weakness; they're simply an integral part of the human experience, of the extraordinary journey to the summit of success. Understanding this is critical to building a support network that fosters resilience, provides help, and celebrates inner strength.

In moments of personal triumph, we often neglect to acknowledge the complex psychological burdens we carry. However, these burdens do not subtract from our achievements. Instead, they add a layer of grit, resilience, and authenticity to the journey.

Our mental health is every bit as significant as our physical health, and the two are intrinsically intertwined. It's time we recognized this. As high achievers, leaders, and trailblazers, we have the potential and the responsibility to bring mental health out of the shadows, and into the limelight.

The Illusory Ideal and The Real Deal

Imagine, if you will, the corridors of power—gleaming corporate towers, ivy league board rooms, state-of-the-art medical facilities. This 'is the stage where our high achievers perform. They are the actors in a narrative guided by action, ambition, and unprecedented accomplishments. The spotlight rarely dims, and their audience is global.

From the glossy pages of newsletters to the penetrating lens of the media, they are the embodiment of success and power. We see honed physiques, tailored suits, glowing smiles, and the aura of control that seems perpetually present—a blueprint of perfection we aspire to replicate, a standard we measure ourselves against.

As spectators in this highly choreographed performance, we perceive only what the curtain permits. The final act of triumph after a conflict, the smooth execution after hours of practice, the calm demeanor despite the storm brewing underneath—an illusion contrived for our consumption.

While we marvel at the strength, resilience, and tenacity embodied by these achievers, we see the manifestation of their skills and strengths, not the agonizing journey it took to cultivate them. We experience the celebration, not the struggle. We see the victor, never the contender. We become acquainted with the persona, but not the person.

What remains unseen are the hours of painstaking effort, the crushing self-doubts, the daily battles with their own minds. The challenges they shoulder are much like an iceberg—only a small portion visible, while the vast majority remains submerged beneath the surface, in the shadows of the unknown.

This illusion of perfection, however, is nothing more than a smokescreen, a polished exterior that hides the human being within. Beneath the surface, the reality of the high achiever's life unfurls, marked by long hours, unyielding expectations, and the toll they take on mental health.

The glittering lure of success can be dangerously deceptive. When we witness only the achievements, we inadvertently downplay the grueling work, the painstaking sacrifices, and the toll it takes on the mind and soul. This illusory scenario creates an unsustainable reality—a reality that compels us to hide our struggles, to mask our anxieties, to ignore our fears in order to maintain the façade of triumph.

My uncle's life was a testament to this illusory ideal. His prestigious medical degree, his successful practice, his picture-perfect family—all of these created an image of flawless success. But behind this façade was a man struggling with the weight of expectations, cultural isolation, and a deepening depression that went unnoticed and untreated.

Let's remember to honor the very human struggles co-existing with these unparalleled achievements. Every high achiever is, foremost, a person, carrying burdens just as heavy and daunting as their successes are significant and bright. Underneath the shining armor of accomplishment resides a heart that beats erratically under stress, a mind that races with worry, a soul yearning for relief.

However, the journey does not end here. The path to personal development becomes clearer as we learn to value not just the sheen of success, but also the authentic grit, the real struggles, and the genuine courage it takes to win battles, both seen and unseen.

By shifting our lens, we can behold the whole picture—the human behind the high achiever, the employee behind the executive, the person behind the persona. As we embark on this exploration, we encourage not just them, but everyone, to step out of the shadows, away from the illusions, and into the empowering landscape of personal growth and accepting mental health struggles.

Our converging paths in the following parts of this journey will serve as a reminder that beneath the external glitter of success lie real stories, authentic emotions, and personal battles. It's time we reflected on them, embraced them, and ultimately, found strength in them. Echoing the unmistakable truth that even in their imperfection, we're not alone. Because, after all, perfection is not a prerequisite for extraordinary, and flaws not incompatible with formidable. Our next step is to look deeper into the power of vulnerability and our journey to wield it as our strength.

Affirming Inner Strength and Courage: From Wounded Survivors to Victorious Warriors

As we tread the path of understanding to action, there's a metamorphosis that unfolds within us. The burdens we carried silently become our badges of honor. In wrestling with our mental health challenges, we bring forth inner strength and courage that perhaps we weren't aware we possessed. Isn't it an interesting paradox that in our struggles, we find the incredible strength of our spirit.

This strength, this resilience, is not something we conjure up overnight. It's the culmination of our journey so far—the vulnerability we've embraced, the stigma we've challenged, the daily habits we've culti-vated, the stories we've shared, and the leaps of faith we've taken.

For a moment, let's take a pause to savor this realization. Breathe in. Breathe out. Become aware of the air filling your lungs. Feel your heart beating staunchly inside your chest. Now is the time to affirm:

"I am more than my struggles. I am a blend of strength, resilience, and courage. My mental health battles do not define me but refine me. I am ready to embrace my authentic self for a fulfilling life ahead."

This statement is not just an affirmation. It's a rallying cry, resound-ing with the unstoppable spirit of a warrior. It captures the essence of our endeavors, celebrates the battles we've fought, and announces our readiness for future challenges.

Yes, mental health issues can feel like a sprawling maze, filled with deceptive turns and blind corners. But remember, every venture into this labyrinth polishes our grit, sharpens our minds, and illuminates our path. Each experience is a stepping stone leading us towards acceptance and recovery. Each struggle encountered is a step towards a celebration of life that embraces imperfections and finds joy in personal growth.

As we stand at this juncture, let's vow to continue fostering re-silience, courage, and strength. Learning, growing, and winning our mental battles isn't a race—it's a lifelong journey.

There are still layers to unravel and secrets to discover in our inner sanctuary. This exploration calls for resilience, a quiet kind of courage that allows high achievers to rise to challenges, bounce back from set-backs, and transform stress into a catalyst for growth. The quest isn't over yet; we're just getting started.

The journey ahead takes us further into the untapped crevices and unexplored terrains of our minds. A tranquil sanctuary awaits us, filled with the secret strategies to manage stress and cultivate inner resilience —strategies that you, as high-achievers, can adopt to not just survive but thrive in the face of trials.

The sanctuary offers shelter and solace. It's a place for rejuvenation and reflection. A place where we can rest, refuel, and prepare for our next adventure. Are we ready to explore it?

With resilience coursing through our veins, courage as our compass, and strength as our guide, let's step into the sanctuary. Remember, the journey continues for us to claim not just success, but a life that is deeply fulfilling, authentic, and happy.

The sanctuary doors are opening. Are we ready to step in? Climbing the ladder of professional success is one thing, and we've mastered it. Now, let's conquer the steps to mental wellness, inner peace, and personal satisfaction. The challenge stands—do we dare to accept?

2

⧯

The High-Achiever's Sanctuary: Unraveling the Secret to Stress Management and Inner Resilience

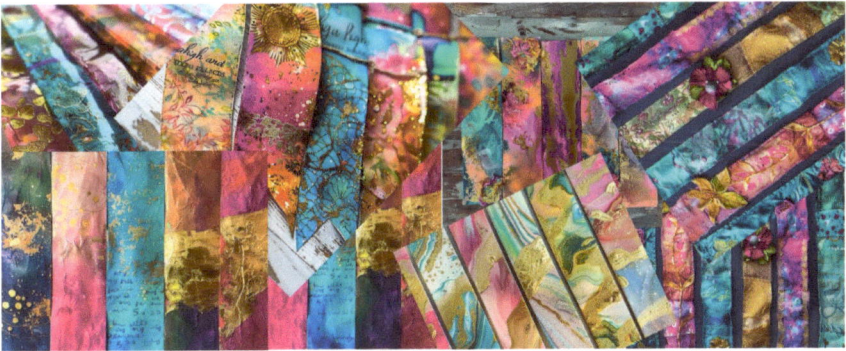

"Harness thy stress, transform it into thy resolute strength; 'tis the true sanctuary of the high-achiever."

When we enter the gleaming structures of bustling cities, we often find the high achievers - respected, admired, and often leading the pack in their respective worlds. Commanding boardrooms, innovating businesses, and charting out strategic directions for some of the world's most notable corporations, they are modern-day gladiators thriving amidst high-pressure environments. Yet, these heavenly heights often accompany overwhelming stress, an invisible, relentless adversary that can cast a formidable shadow over their brightly burning accomplishments.

Yet, here's the secret. Stress, that relentless adversary, can also be your most resilient conduit to extraordinary strength and personal growth. Yes, the bustling battlefield can also be your serene sanctuary. You might be wondering how that's even possible.

The answer lay hidden in plain sight within the principle that underpins this chapter: Harness thy stress, transform it into thy resolute strength; 'tis the true sanctuary of the high-achiever.

This principle asserts that mastering stress, rather than merely combating it, is the underlying bedrock of high achievement and enduring resilience. It unveils the profound transformation in perspective: viewing stress, not as an undermining adversary but a resilient ally.

Imagine transforming that brute, unyielding stress into enduring strength, resilience, and incredible success. Imagine it, not as a villain of your story, but as a guide into the heart of your true potential. Picture it educating you, evolving you, and equipping you to journey towards a profound sense of personal fulfillment and joy. All this whilst you still enjoy and contribute proactively to your high-achieving lifestyle.

With this principle as the true north of our conversation, the ensuing sections of this chapter will accompany your journey from understanding the manifestations of stress to discovering its root causes. From there, you'll learn to thrive amidst the chaos, using stress as a profound catalyst for growth. You'll recognize stress symptoms, signs, and triggers with newfound insight, even as you begin to develop effective strategies for managing this formidable force.

This chapter is a promise to you. A promise of empowerment and enlightenment, wrapped in a tone that is motivational, practical, enlightening, fearless, and most of all, fun. Embarking on this journey of navigating your life with a perspective shift could inspire you to live a deeply fulfilling life, cherishing moments with loved ones and finding happiness beyond professional success. You'll realize that stress is not as insurmountable as it seems. Instead, it can be sculpted into a source of strength that not only endures, but thrives.

With unstoppable resolve, relentless determination, and armed with actionable insights from this chapter, you are set to craft your story of transforming stress into strength - crafting a life that is not only successful but also deeply fulfilling. As we transition into the first section of this chapter, prepare to explore the paradoxical nature of success, a journey of triumphing over and tripping over stress.

Prepare to explore mapping the maze of the high-achievers' world, where glittering success and formidable stress often walk hand in hand. So, take a deep breath, keep the principle of transforming stress into enduring strength in mind, and journey with me into this empowering sanctuary.

The Dichotomy of Success: Triumphing Over and Tripping Over Stress

There is perhaps no adventure more exhilarating or fulfilling as that of the relentless climb to success. It's a journey that amasses abundant laurels yet thrusts equally colossal stresses upon the high-achievers who tread it. For those in their shoes, stress becomes a paradox - a trigger of both their triumph and their tribulations.

To the uninitiated, it might seem as though high-achievers don the guise of modern-day gladiators, brandishing their suits and power ties against the corporate arena's challenges. However, unbeknownst to onlookers, the arenas they conquer each day are not only filled with business adversaries but also teeming with an invisible rival—overwhelming stress.

Unresolved stress, like an unnoticed sand grain in an oyster, can wreak havoc if left unchecked. It can transform from a minor irritant into a debilitating issue, casting a formidable shadow over one's outwardly glittering success. However, unlike the oyster, who might turn an unwelcome grain of sand into a precious pearl, high-achievers often grapple with transforming their stress into a valuable asset. Instead, the relentless mental turmoil they endure, silently erodes their happiness, fulfillment, and often, their health - a heavy price to pay for their clamorous success.

Yet, beneath these waves of adversity, an undercurrent of transformation awaits discovery. The soaring heights of success and the plunging abyss of stress, though seemingly paradoxical, are uniquely connected. They are two sides of the same coin. As high-achievers, the challenge lies in mastering this dichotomy - to triumph over stress while you trip over it, to transmute it into the strong alloy that fortifies your climb to success.

Stress, when perceived and handled astutely, can be harnessed into a force that propels you towards personal growth and resilience, much like the pearl created from an irksome grain of sand. It is an invitation to a profound self-dialogue, to introspect deeper into your psyche. Are you running away from stress or learning from it? Are you letting it suffocate your potential or sculpt it?

Unseen to many, high achievers often use their stress as an impetus to surmount challenges and elevate their successes. Not by negating stress, but by engaging with it constructively. By acknowledging it as an integral, albeit uncomfortable, part of their life narrative. By gleaning insights from its lessons, they mold stress into a catalyst for tremendous personal and professional growth.

Triumphing over stress doesn't necessarily imply eradicating it. Rather, it signifies using it as a stepping stone rather than a stumbling block. It is an invitation to redirect the overpowering energy of stress towards enhancing mental strength and resilience. And this, dear reader, forms the crux of our exploration within this section.

Let's look into this dichotomy of success, and prepare to redefine your perception of stress. Understand its manifestation and navigate its complexities. You'll discover how to dance gracefully with stress and transform it into your secret ally in the journey towards achieving your peak potential. Buckle up and join me on this transformative journey into the heart of your stress, right into the birthplace of pearls.

The Invisible Chains: Understanding the Manifestations of Stress

As high achievers grapple with the daily rigors of their personal and professional lives, stress coils around them like invisible chains, holding them hostage in their own landscapes of success. To an observer, these chains remain unseen, shrouded by the glamorous exterior of success and accomplishment. Yet, for the individuals embroiled within them, they weigh heavy and tight.

Stress, akin to an uninvited guest, forcefully inserts itself into all aspects of life. It doesn't discriminate, entangling the mental, physical, and emotional selves. Like a shapeshifter, it takes varying forms - from restlessness, anxiety, irritability, and insomnia to diminished concentration, appetite fluctuations, lethargy, and beyond.

But here's the enlightening facet. While physical symptoms are often more obvious and impossible to ignore, the mental manifestations of stress are undeniably more profound and consequential. Feelings of being overwhelmed, persistent worrying, difficulty concentrating, and negative thinking patterns are often warning flags of stress becoming a mental ordeal.

Moreover, in some cases, the shadow of overwhelming stress casts darkness over one's self-perceptions, manifesting into insecurities around self-esteem and body image concerns. Here, the struggle intensifies as stress warps the mirror of self-view, leading individuals to distort and criticize their physical appearance in a sea of negative self-talk and body dissatisfaction.

The relentless pursuit of perfection, which often fuels the success of high-achievers, further adds momentum to the domino effect of stress manifestations. The constant striving to meet exceedingly high expectations — from oneself and others — reinforces the stress cycle, leading to exhaustion, burnout, and eventually, an emotional collapse.

Recognizing these manifestations of stress is the first step on the journey to managing it skillfully. As Nathaniel Branden once said, "The first step toward change is awareness."

The chains of stress, though invisible, become tangible when seen through the lens of its manifestations. The symptoms we discussed serve as links in this chain - each one interlinked, creating a complex web of responses that affect you mentally, emotionally, and physically. Once we grasp these links, we begin to understand the weight and impact of stress on our lives, thus empowering ourselves to initiate steps towards its strategic management.

Dear reader, as we immerse deeper into the invisible chains of stress, take a moment to assess your own relationship with stress. Can you identify the links in your chain? How does your stress manifest? When is it most present? Reflection and self-scrutiny are the keys to unlock profound insights into your personal stress narrative. Verily, these insights serve as the compass guiding us along the meandering journey ahead.

Are you, prepared to unearth the root causes of stress? It's in understanding the 'why' behind our stress; we discover the courage to break the chains binding us. Swim with me, dear reader, deeper into the swirling currents of your stress manifestations, towards the peace lying at your journey's end.

Thriving Amidst the Chaos: Stress as a Catalyst for Growth

Stress. A five-letter word that often comes laden with negative connotations, but what if we reimagine stress as an opportunity, as a catalyst for growth rather than a deterrent? At first, it may seem like a pipe dream, conjuring up images of high-achievers, like you, thriving amidst mounting pressure. Yet, it is precisely in this paradox that the magic unfolds. As we step foot into this segment, we aim to shatter the illusion of stress as a villain and rather grace it as a concealed companion on the journey to personal success.

Imagine stress as a mightily flowing river, uninterrupted and chaotically beautiful. It rushes past with immense force, carving its path through mountains and plains alike. High-achievers often find themselves in the heart of this river, battling the currents, trying to keep afloat.

But think for a moment — what if the same energy that fueled the violent currents could help you navigate through them, not merely to stay afloat, but to stride forth confidently? That's the transformational power we're unearthing today – harnessing stress as a catalyst for growth.

Embrace the mantra: Stress makes you resilient. Like Robert H. Schuller rightly said, "Tough times never last, but tough people do". When faced with demanding situations, stress can elicit a powerful response from within, forcing you to dig deep into your reservoirs of strength and resilience. It is in such throbbing beats of adversity that most high-achievers find the rhythm of their greatest growth.

Stress also polishes your problem-solving skills. As you constantly engage with challenging situations, you strengthen your ability to think on your feet, make swift decisions, and navigate complexities with aplomb. Over time, the daunting mountains of stress morph into stepping stones, fostering an improvement in cognitive flexibility, creativity, and determination.

Moreover, stress can be a potent motivator, spurring you into action. It can nudge you out of inertia, trigger productive behaviors, and kindle a sense of urgency essential to meet your goals. Experiencing stress is often an indication that you are pushing boundaries, exploring uncharted territories, and inching closer to your peak potential.

Now, the question beckons – how do we initiate this transformation; how do we morph stress from an overwhelming force into a propellant that fuels growth?

The key, dear reader, lies in shifting the perspective from perceiving stress as a foe to embracing it as an ally. It involves calculatedly engaging with stress, understanding its dynamics, and finally redirecting its immense energy towards productive outcomes.

In the course of our exploration, we've identified the manifestations of stress and acknowledged its potent presence in your lives. Now, enlightened and fortified with a new outlook, we are equipped to descend deeper, to unearth the roots of our personal stress.

As we continue our exploration, keep in mind that the journey to understanding and managing stress doesn't end here. In fact, we've only just started unraveling the mystery that is stress— understanding its manifestations was just a stepping stone. Every step we take provides further insight leading us towards greater mastery over this complex yet transformative force in our lives. So, hold on with me, dear reader, as we dive deeper into the 'why' of our stress, embarking on yet another enlightening chapter in this journey to stress mastery and inner resilience. Shall we?

Beyond the Surface: Discovering the Root Causes of Stress

In the musical harmonies of life, each note carries its unique rhythm, creating a synchronized melody. Similarly, stress isn't born in isolation. It's an intricate tapestry woven with threads of various experiences, underlying beliefs, societal conditioning, and personal drivers. To conquer stress truly, it isn't enough to understand its manifestations and transform it into a catalyst for growth. Indeed, this is a monumental leap. Yet, to fully skew the scales in our favor, we need to climb deeper, to untangle the roots of our personal stress triggers.

Imagine an enormous, majestic oak tree representing stress. Its leaves swaying in the breeze signify its outward manifestations, while the trunk and sturdy branches epitomize strength and resilience. Thriving amidst chaos, we've accepted and harnessed these tangible elements of stress. Now, it's time to dig deeper, beneath the verdant foliage, into the vast network of roots making this giant oak—or stress—stand tall.

These roots symbolize a myriad of factors, ranging from perceived burdens of expectations, self-imposed pressures, societal norms, to personal fears, that fabricate the colossal structure of stress. As high achievers, you are likely to find threads of perfectionism, fear of failure, imposter syndrome, or relentless striving for success in your roots, each of which contributes to your unique "stress DNA."

Expectations come in as a significant driving root. We're programmed from an early age to meet the societal norms and familial standards set for us. The benchmarks aren't necessarily negative in themselves, but obsessively aiming to meet or exceed them without a moment's pause transforms a positive drive into a chronic stress source.

Likewise, high achievers often set extraordinarily high standards for themselves. Fueled by perfectionism, this self-imposed pressure of "never good enough" can become a root cause for constant stress. Constantly pushing boundaries and the pursuit of a flawless work-life balance can make the scale wobble, inflating the stress balloon more.

Underlying fears, too, nurture the root system of stress. Fear of failure, the dread of not living up to others' expectations, or even the anxiety of success can create a state of continuous stress, affecting one's self-esteem and mental peace.

Understanding these underlying threads is pivotal because every battle won against stress is a victory over these root causes that fuel it. But digging up these roots is not an attempt to eradicate them. On the contrary, it's about understanding their influence, embracing them, and learning to maneuver around them.

As we tread this enlightening path together, begin introspecting about your root causes of stress. Jot them down, observe them, reflect on them. This exploration, although challenging, unravels hidden truths about your unique experiences with stress.

Remember, the power to manage your stress resides within you. It lies in understanding that stress roots don't define you but enlighten you about the 'what' and 'why' of your stress. This understanding arms us with the ammunition needed to tackle it tactically, to craft a map for strategic stress management.

This excavation is just another layer in the onion of stress. Extraction, understanding, and management come hand in hand, setting the stage for you to redefine your relationship with stress. Let's dig deeper, strive harder, and gather more tools for your arsenal against stress. Step into the world of strategic stress management practices as we continue our journey, ready to manage stress with conviction and steadfastness. Together, we're one step closer to mastering stress and enjoying the symphony of life sans the discordant notes of stress. Let's stride forward with heads held high and hearts alight with purpose on this journey towards true stress mastery and inner resilience.

The High-Achiever's Blueprint: Effective Strategies for Stress Management

Having unmasked the hidden faces of stress and dissected its roots and impacts, the transformative journey towards managing stress begins. Stress, much like formidable opponents we encounter, meets a valiant contender in the strategies we adopt to restrict its engulfing hold over us. In the realm of high-achievers––where you hail from––these strategies must mirror the dynamism, versatility, and mindfulness inherent in your lives.

Let's envision this as crafting a highly conducive sanctuary, specifically designed to combat your unique stress patterns. Just as an architect delineates spaces as per functionality and aesthetics while keeping the inhabitants in mind, we too will blueprint a strategy with your individual proclivities at its core.

Our first building block in this blueprint is 'Awareness'. Merely acknowledging stress and its root causes isn't enough when we aim to manage it effectively. Cultivating an intimate awareness of personal triggers, reactions, and behaviors associated with stress paves the path to stress management.

Breathing deeply, let us then add the pillar of 'Mindfulness'. A skill that may seem elusive in the race against ticking clocks, but absolute mindfulness can be your secret weapon against stress. Carve out moments to be completely present, free from the constant need to rush, harbor expectations, or meet standards. Be it through meditation, mindful eating, or even a simple walk in the park, allow your senses to imbibe your experiences fully.

Resilience - is our next component. The realization that a change in perspective can transform mountains into molehills is a stepping stone to building resilience. Remember, "tough times never last, but tough people do?" Letting challenges propel us forward instead of holding us back fortifies our ability to withstand stress.

Further fortifying our blueprint, we embed 'Self-care' solidly into the concoction. No, it's not indulgent; it's a necessity. From ensuring a proper sleep schedule, nutritious diet, regular exercise to setting boundaries, prioritizing 'me' time, and allowing moments of joy, an adequately cared-for you is a better armed you against stress.

Finally, 'Seeking Support' forms the roof of our sanctuary. There's an empowering beauty in vulnerability and seeking help when needed. Surround yourself with positive relationships, consider professional help if needed, lean on faith and spirituality, and participate in social activities that enhance well-being.

In crafting this blueprint, you're building not just a sanctuary against stress, but a nourishing environment facilitating growth, happiness, and personal success. Remember, it's your sanctuary, customized and crafted with love, determination, and hope.

Now, armed with a sound blueprint, we are prepared to put these strategies into practice. It's not about instant transformations, it's about persistent, gradual changes leading to monumental shifts in managing stress.

As we take a moment to appreciate the growth and insights gleaned so far, we move forward into the affirmation of strength and triumph. It's time to look stress in the eye and declare,

"I am the architect of my life; I transform my stress into strength, channeling it to fuel my growth and resilience. My stress doesn't control me, I control it."

Ready to carry this affirmation in your heart, we march ahead, breaking free from the chains of stress, eager to master and redefine our relationship with the defining paradox of today's age – stress. So, gear up to step into the resilience battleground, where we sculpt our stress into our ally and emerge more powerful than ever, renewed in our purpose and resolve.

The Resilient Battleground: Affirmation of Strength and Triumph

As we unfurl the final chapter in the stress saga, admire how far you've journeyed. You've not only identified, accepted, and understood the mighty presence of stress in your life, but trod the path towards managing it effectively. Applaud your strength for challenging the long-held belief that high levels of stress are a by-product of success. Now, arriving at the inflection point of this journey, it is time to celebrate you.

Our inscription in the sands of time is colored by our experiences, strengths, vulnerabilities, and triumphs. It is punctuated by the infusion of change and the audacity to seek that change. Among these myriad colors, the most vibrant hue is your resilience. Stand tall, resonating in the illumination of your inner strength, in the glow of your triumph over adversity.

Now, in the silence that follows the storm, brace yourself to utter the declaration of victory. Close your eyes and let the affirmation sink deep into your being:

"I am the architect of my life; I transform my stress into strength, channeling it to fuel my growth and resilience. My stress doesn't control me, I control it."

This affirmation is not merely a collection of words but a taproot vitalizing your resilience against stress. It is your talisman, carved by your vulnerable moments, your victories, your bouts of courage, and your fearlessness. It is your testament of unwavering faith, your ode to resilience, your proclamation of triumph.

You are not simply battling stress; you are crafting a narrative of resilience. You are not merely a high achiever veiled behind success; you are the embodiment of the resilience that successes and failures forge.

As we bid adieu to the battle against stress, remember — the fierce wars you wage against your demons mold your spirit into an unassailable fortress. Each daunting endeavor strengthens your resilience. Each challenge makes you more formidable. Each setback lights the beacon of wisdom brighter.

You have peered into the heart of your stress, acknowledged its roots, recognized its manifestations, and crafted a sanctuary against it. Now, armored with a blueprint to combat it and a powerful affirmation in your heart, you have stepped out, triumphant, onto the resilient battleground.

Remember, your confrontation with stress isn't a destination but a journey — one that you will embrace and steer, armed with resilience, wisdom, and emotional grit. Let this journey illuminate your path and reinforce your faith in your ability to convert stress into a strength.

With heads held high and hearts aglow with the affirmation, we bring this exploration to a close only to transition into a new dawn. A horizon where we reinvent, rediscover, and redefine the relationship with the inevitable companion of our modern lives – stress. So, let's stride forward, fueled by the rhythm of resilience, into the new era of life mastery!

3

Personal Grounding: Cultivating Mental Fortitude in Power-Driven Lifestyles

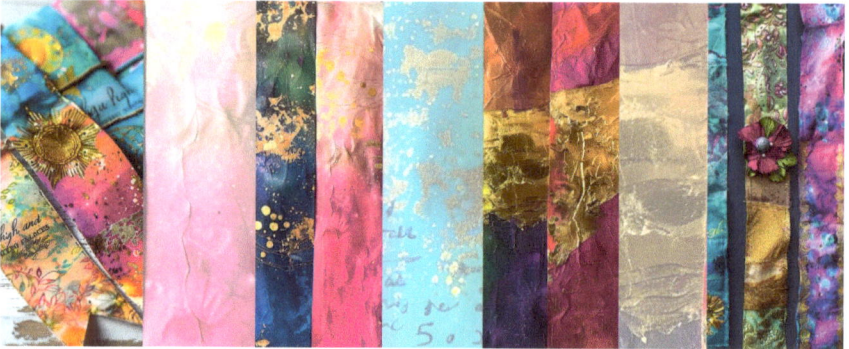

"In the fortress of self, resilience is the architect, vulnerability the cornerstone, and mental fortitude the invincible structure."

The pulse of the city beats beneath your feet as you stand amidst the towering skyscrapers, emblems of your professional conquests. Success. Power. These are the triumphant melodies woven into the very fabric of your life, a testament to the remarkable heights you've scaled in the professional landscape. You, the corporate titans, the spearheads of multibillion-dollar institutions, the trailblazers in your respective domains, are embodiments of determination and resilience. And yet, amidst the applause and admiration, you find yourself in a silent battle with invisible foes – mental health issues.

Beneath the glimmering armor of achievement, you grapple with stress, addiction, self-esteem issues, body image concerns, depression, or anxiety. Balancing high-stakes roles and parenthood, your life is a juggling act under a harsh spotlight, each move scrutinized, each misstep, magnified. This intricate dance has led to the uninvited arrival of invisible adversaries that threaten to topple your world just as swiftly as you've built it.

This chapter is an empowering call to arms for those caught in the grips of these silent battles, those aspiring for a life that is celebrated and not just tolerated. Your journey toward happiness and fulfillment beyond professional success begins here.

Our quest starts with a vital principle, a cornerstone in the edifice of mental resilience - "In the fortress of self, resilience is the architect, vulnerability the cornerstone, and mental fortitude the invincible structure." It signifies the critical balance of recognizing your struggles and harnessing resilience to build an unshakable mental fortress. Each word in this principle mirrors a steppingstone towards personal grounding and inner strength in the face of adversity.

We begin by unmasking the illusion of invulnerability often adorned by high achievers. You'll explore the crucial role of acknowledging emotional vulnerability and embrace it as your liaison in cultivating resilience. The subsequent sections are dedicated to the methodical construction of your mental fortress, a sanctuary built on self-confidence, emotional regulation, and resilience.

This chapter is an ode to the fortress within each of you, a testament to your capacity for resilience and vulnerability, and the valor of your mental fortitude. Each section is tailored as a potent tool in your arsenal, each lesson a steppingstone towards the precipice of self-discovery, self-belief, resilience, and emotional intelligence.

The promise this chapter holds for you is profound and transformative. You will embark on a journey of introspection, moving into your inner recesses, confront your vulnerabilities, and emerge with an invincible mental structure that can weather all storms.

Don't just survive these tumultuous waves; learn to navigate them skillfully, leveraging each crest and trough to propel you towards your triumphs. Each challenge you face will no longer be a stumbling block but a stepping stone, a battlefield that morphs into a platform for victory.

The transformation you'll experience in this chapter is akin to constructing an architectural marvel, brick by brick, with resilience as the architect and vulnerability as the cornerstone. Bereft of these elements, the fortress of self-risks crumbles in the face of adversities.

So dear readers, as we unravel this enticing narrative of mental fortitude, let the promise of transformation ignite a spark of anticipation within. Remember, this journey isn't a sprint but a marathon, a progressive endeavor of building personal grounding. So let's lace up for the transformational journey toward cultivating mental fortitude in this challenging yet rewarding path of power-driven lifestyles.

The Veil of Invulnerability: Embracing Vulnerability to Forge Resilience

As the key holders of empires, the titans of industries, you walk with an assurance that is both admired and expected. You are the actors cast in the roles of invincible gladiators, capable of slaying dragons and scaling heights unfathomable to the regular populace. You are not the harbingers of weakness; you are the paragons of strength, capability, and resilience. And yet, there's an unseen world within you that craves for acknowledgment—the world known as vulnerability.

The specter of vulnerability is something many stalwarts of success shun, considering it akin to a chink in their impenetrable armor. However, believe me when I say this, dear readers, your vulnerability is not your weakness. It is your unrecognized strength. It's high time we shed the misconception that vulnerability means giving in to your weaknesses. That's far from the truth. Instead, it's about having the audacity to acknowledge your struggles and channeling this self-awareness into a force that propels you forward.

Consider vulnerability as the unchartered territory that holds the key to your most profound personal growth. It's akin to a seed that requires darkness to break open and release its life force, and in that process, a formidable tree of self-awareness and resilience sprouts.

Think back on the times when the towering skyscrapers seemed to weigh you down, or the responsibilities threatened to engulf you. Amidst the chaos of board meetings, financial deadlines, and parental demands, have you been kind enough to ask yourself how you're feeling? Have you ever accepted that it's okay to feel overwhelmed, stressed, or anxious? That's where the initiation of a dialogue with your vulnerability begins.

By suppressing your vulnerability, you build a fortress that shuts out potential growth, learning, and self-realization. This fortress, albeit seemingly resilient, robs you of the strength and clarity that come with navigating the turbulent seas of your emotions and understanding your mental state.

So, as you begin this journey, take this pledge - "I'll not shy away from expressing my true feelings, anxieties, or worries. I'll respect these emotions as part of my existence and allow myself to feel, acknowledge, and understand them. I'll embrace vulnerability as an avenue for building my mental resilience."

This vulnerability is your liaison in cultivating resilience. By acknowledging it, you are setting the first crucial stepping stone in your journey towards building an impregnable mental fortress anchored deep within your psyche. It marks the first stage of honoring your emotional spectrum and harnessing mental strength from the heart of your struggles.

As we transition into the next part of this chapter, I challenge you to shift your perspective. See vulnerability for what it truly is - not a sign of weakness, but a badge of courage. Establish a fresh narrative where vulnerability and authenticity are celebrated and not shunned. Remember, this journey is not a sprint but a marathon, one requiring patience, perseverance, and kindness towards oneself. As we peel back the layers of this veil of invulnerability, I invite you to brace yourself for the journey ahead; a transformative sojourn into fortifying your mental constitution in your power-driven journey.

The Personal Fortress: Constructing Your Mental Bulwark

Having traversed through the realm of vulnerability, bear in mind the wisdom it offers. Vulnerability is your inner self, bearing witness to your thoughts, feelings, and emotions. Shunning it is likened to building a fortress devoid of its core—robust yet hollow, impervious but soulless. Now, we begin probing into creating a sanctuary that reflects your complex, beautiful self—a fortress of mental resilience and fortitude.

In this relentless quest for success, envisage your mind as a fortress. Surrounded by the ramparts built with self-confidence, the watchtowers fortified with emotional regulation, and the drawbridge of resilience that shields you from the adversities and perils that lurk outside. Within the calming illumination of self-awareness, these elements coalesce into an impregnable structure—a testament to your indomitable spirit.

Self-confidence forms the very bedrock of this fortress. Confidence empowers you to rise above self-doubt and skepticism, instead pivoting you to focus on your strengths and capabilities. Your self-belief is not a function of external validation but a burning conviction stemming from within you. By cultivating this self-confidence, your actions echo this belief—a manifestation of your assuredness in your abilities and the path you tread.

However, constructing this fortress is no mean feat—it demands emotional regulation. It involves recognizing and understanding your emotions and managing them productively. Consider a day filled to the brim with crises and confrontations. It is natural to harbor feelings of frustration, anxiety, or despair. Emotional regulation teaches you to navigate these emotional tumults without succumbing to them, a trait as vital as the walls furnishing your fortress.

Yet, the most robust of fortresses would crumble without the drawbridge of resilience. Picture every setback, every failure, and every disappointment as a cannonball aimed at your fortress. Without resilience, your fortress would succumb to the onslaught and eventually shatter. However, resilience empowers you to rebound from these adversities, reinforcing and fortifying your fortress after every attack.

Let's store this wisdom in the treasure chest of our newfound fortress. Suppressing struggles creates a hollow fortress, devoid of its essence. Embrace vulnerability and recognize its potential as a stepping stone towards building your sturdy, richly adorned fortress of mental fortitude. In this fortress, let self-confidence be the foundation, emotional regulation be the walls, and resilience, the drawbridge warding off adversities.

As we progress from this introspective exploration, let's carry forth the tools and wisdom acquired. Firm in our resolve, let's embark on the meticulous task of building this fortress in the upcoming landscape of our quest.

Remember, your mental fortress is not merely a symbol of strength. It is the profound embodiment of your personal journey, experiences, and growth. As we transition further into this quest, empowering ourselves with the pillars of mental strength, the emblem of our unique individuality awaits to cement a resilient fortress in the windswept landscapes of our minds.

Pillars of Power: Self-Belief, Resilience and Emotional Intelligence

A fortress, irrespective of its robust construct, cannot hold its stand without reinforced pillars. Similarly, a firm mental fortitude relies on the strength of some critical inner pillars; self-belief, resilience, and emotional intelligence.

Picture your self-belief as the first pillar that holds your mental fortress upright. It is this belief that fuels your pursuit of success, even in the face of resistance. Self-belief envelops you in a protective shell, guarding you in times of self-doubt, conflict, and criticism. It's your lifeline in the whirlpool of life, letting you emerge resolute and unscathed. Let self-belief be your armor in the battlefield of life, transforming potential defeats into empowering victories.

Next appears the resilient pillar, the epitome of tenacity and endurance. Resilience is crucial in facing the challenges hurled at your fortress. Think of resilience as the Phoenix, rising and re-emerging from the ashes of setback, stronger and fiercer! It equips you to bounce back, enabling you to rebuild parts of your fort that crumble under the weight of adversities. Remember, every scar makes your fortress resilient and adds to the stories etched in your walls.

Emotional intelligence, the third pillar, plays a significant role in developing mental fortitude. It empowers you to understand, interpret, and manage both your emotions and those of others. Imagine a bustling market, swirling with different voices. Emotional intelligence is your ability to discern valuable information amidst this cacophony and connect with people's unique stories and perspectives. Emotional intelligence within your fortress increases your capacity for empathy and develops your interpersonal skills.

The foundation has been laid, and the walls erected. Our fortress now stands with its three robust pillars- the self-belief that fuels our action, the resilience that guards us from adversities, and the emotional intelligence that enhances our relationship with the world.

As our exploration of the fortress deepens, take a moment to appreciate these pillars of strength you've painstakingly built. Understand their role and their synergy in reinforcing your mental fortress. Embrace the harmony created by self-belief, resilience, and emotional intelligence, marking a crucial milestone in your exploration.

As we step into the next corridor of this fortress that we've been building, keep in mind that our journey is as unique as ourselves. While we navigate the battleground of life and triumph, remember that our struggles and fears are not shackles but stepping stones toward forti-tude. As we go deeper into the art of crafting mental fortitude, let's prepare ourselves for the potential battles and expected triumphs that lie ahead on our journey toward personal growth.

Frame of Fortitude: From Battles to Triumphs

Gazing upon our familiar fortress, recognize the trials, struggles, and triumphs engraved into its structure. The path to a fortified mind is rife with battles and victories alike. Each strife encountered and each victory achieved are integral aspects of this journey.

Consider the battlefield of life; it is here where our mental fortitude is truly put to the test. Picture the moments when stress, doubt, and fear sought to breach the fortress walls. Remember the inner turmoil, the whispers of uncertainty and the gusts of distress threatening to leave your fortitude in ruins. Every wrinkle etched into the fortress's facade tells tales of the challenges faced—the battles fought within these walls.

A profound realization dawns amidst these battles; challenges are not obstacles but opportunities—opportunities that can fan the embers of potential into flames of triumph. With self-belief as our guide, resil-ience as our shield, and emotional intelligence as our compass, we can navigate the stormy seas of adversity to find the shores of victory. Each setback, each defeat is but a stepping-stone leading towards the crest of triumph.

Visualize the moments of resilience that propelled you past these battles. The rise from the ashes of defeat, the strength harnessed from every challenge, every moment when resilience fortified the fortress's ramparts. Cherish these victories, for they embody the spirit of over-coming—of transforming battles into triumphs. Remember, each battle is merely a prologue, setting the stage for emerging victories.

Now, let's walk towards the Triumph Fort—the symbolic representation of victory. Carved into its imposing stone walls, are the stories of adversities transformed into triumph. Each character gracing this fort is a testament to an individual's resilience, perseverance, and determination. A triumphant reminder of how far one has walked on the journey towards cultivating mental fortitude.

The journey through this Triumph Fort is an empowering testament to the transformative power of perspective. It reveals how viewing adversities not as setbacks but as catalysts for fortitude can shift our path from struggle to victory. It illuminates the inherent potential in every challenge and encourages us to embrace, not evade life's battles.

As we go deeper into the art of crafting mental fortitude, let's embody this power of transforming adversities into stepping stones to success. Clutch this empowering perspective tightly, looking at the practical, tangible, and actionable steps that would lead to the architecting of our mental fortress—a fortress cemented with battles, adorned with triumphs, and aglow with resilience. Remember, the journey towards fortitude is not a series of battles but a saga of transformation—from combating adversities to celebrating victories, from addressing challenges to architecting an indomitable mental fortress in the windswept landscapes of our minds.

Blueprint of the Mind: Shaping Your Mental Fortitude Strategy

Enlightening tales of battles and victories adorn the walls of our mental fortress—the powerful, vivid reminders of the transformative journey we've taken thus far. With this awareness of our resilience, the time has come to put an action plan into place—the Blueprint of the Mind—which would help us maneuver the labyrinth of mental fortitude with purposeful strides.

Our journey towards cultivating mental fortitude is a purposeful navigation through the battlefield of life. It's time to equip ourselves with practical, tangible, and actionable tools to weather the storms of our existence with grace and fortitude. Think of these tools as the architect's instruments, each of them crucial to designing the blueprint of your mental fortitude strategy.

Begin with setting clear and personalized goals. Our goals could range from enhancing our emotional intelligence, strengthening our self-belief, to developing superior resilience. They act as the guiding stars that light our path toward an unshaken mental fortitude. Remember, the goals must reflect your unique journey, resonating with your struggles, victories, and aspirations.

Next, focus on mental conditioning. Like a seasoned warrior gearing up for battle, practice conducting regular mental exercises to prepare for inevitable struggles. Carve out time for mindfulness, gratitude practices, reflection, or even therapeutic hobbies that foster emotional stability and peace. This discipline of mental conditioning adjusts the very dimensions of your fortress, heightening the walls and sharpening the towers.

As your Blueprint expands, make room for emotional regulation—a vital tool to harness emotional intelligence. Remember the bustling market analogy we discussed? Mastering your emotions amidst the highs and lows of life is akin to discerning valuable information within the chaos. Techniques such as meditation, journaling, or deep-breathing exercises can assist in managing emotional highs and lows.

Lastly, concentrate on strengthening resilience. We've already seen how a resilient mindset can turn battles into triumphs. Incorporate practices that promote resilience, such as facing fears, cultivating optimism, or fostering problem-solving skills.

As we wrap up our architect's plan, allow yourself to experience a cascade of emotions—an empowering blend of anticipation, excitement, thrill, even a little fear. But above all, feel an overwhelming sense of determination, as if the weight of the fortress's stones is a reassuring pat on the back, gently whispering, 'You've got this.'

And remember, the beauty of this Blueprint lies in its perpetual evolution. It is not a rigid document, but rather a living, breathing guide that grows with each step you take in this transformative journey. Every challenge encountered, every victory achieved, every goal realized - they all leave an imprint on this plan, molding it into a reflection of your ever-evolving journey towards mental fortitude.

This strategy will be your blueprint, your roadmap to embracing not just the triumphs but also the trials along the way. As we step into the next corridor of our journey, we move beyond the theoretical understanding of mental strength towards a tangible, practical realization of fortitude. It's about installing the final piece of our grand fortress puzzle: a triumphant declaration of reclaiming power through inner resilience. It's time to embrace the architect within and finesse the art of erecting our fortress of mental fortitude. We march forward, not just as warriors, but as architects, builders, and wielders of our destiny.

Empowered Proclamation: Reclaiming Your Innate Power through Mental Fortitude

The architect's plans have been drawn out; the walls of the fortress fortified. The blueprints of your mind have been meticulously designed, etched with the tales of battles, victories, and transformative lessons. Now it's time to stand tall amidst these battlements of resilience, self-belief, and emotional intelligence, to feel the weight of your power, your control, and your capability. This is your triumphant declaration of having reclaimed power through the cultivation of inner resilience.

"No longer is stress my conqueror, it is my prompter. No longer are failures my enemies, they are my teachers. I am not a slave to my mental health issues—they are battles I am equipped to face and equipped to conquer. I am the master architect of my mental fortitude—resilient in face of trials, flexible amidst shifts, and empowered by my unshakeable self-belief. I embrace every facet of my existence, standing resolute, ready to excel in life's throes."

There is power in this affirmation, echoing the essence of all we've discussed about fortifying our minds and lives. It fuels the determination, sparkles the motivation and nurtures the resilience to face the stormy weathers of challenges and mental health battles. This is the mantra that will echo within your mental fortress, its echoes resonating off the sturdy walls of your fortitude.

And so, let it echo, let it resonate, let it become the empowering rhythm of your struggles and victories. Let it serve as a constant reminder of your unwavering potential and power, a testament to your journey and proof of your evolution into a mentally fortified warrior. You are the architect of your destiny, a warrior walking the path of resilience, a navigator setting the sails towards the horizon of mental fortitude.

But remember, this is not the end of the journey but the beginning of a new chapter— a chapter where you will continue to build upon this fortress, strengthening it, expanding it one mindful brick at a time. This fortress lives, breathes, and grows with you, every added stone being a record of your journey—of challenges faced, of victories celebrated.

Now as we close the doors of this mental fortress, it's time to reveal the key that will open the doors to conquering dependencies in high-powered lifestyles. Because precisely like the storms of challenges and mental health battles, dependencies are battles that we are equipped to face and equipped to conquer. Remember, we are warriors walking the path of resilience, navigating the labyrinth of life, one step at a time. And it's time to take the next step into the next chapter of our journey-towards understanding and overcoming dependencies, toward weaving an Addiction Almanac.

4

The Addiction Almanac: A Comprehensive Guide to Understanding and Overcoming Dependencies in High-Powered Lifestyles

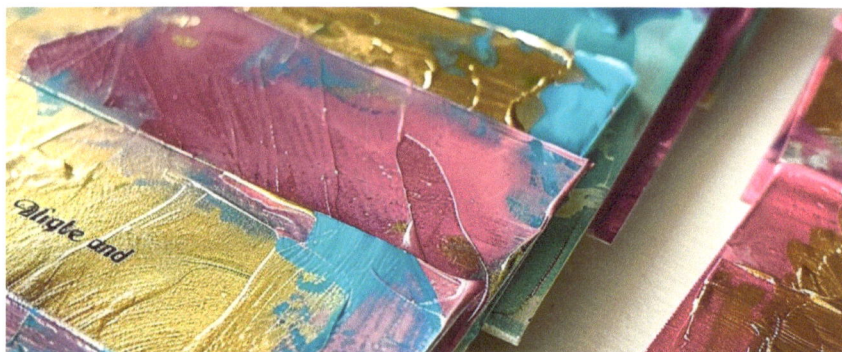

"Mastering the mind, we break free from addiction's chains: to know freedom, we first grasp the cage"

Welcome to a chapter fraught with discovery, an exploration into a topic all-too-familiar with high achievers but seldom discussed aloud. Here we pull back the veil on the silent thief lurking in the lives of the successful world over - Addiction. Surprising, isn't it? But the world of high-powered lifestyles can obscure certain truths, even to the most discerning eyes.

You've climbed the steep summits of success, conquered the demanding terrains of high-pressure professions, weathered the storms of challenges, balancing plates precariously between family obligations and professional commitments. These victories bear witness to your strength, resilience, fortitude, and the relentless pursuit of your dreams. Yet, there's a mysterious trap hidden amidst your accomplishments, one that can weave an intricate web around your life, unnoticed. Addiction.

Addiction, through this chapter, will no longer merely stand for hard substances misused; it will unfold as behavioral dependencies, habits formed under pressure, stress, and the relentless desire to maintain stride in the race of high-powered, success-driven lifestyles. The shackles of this hidden dependency can creep into your life disguised as intricate patterns and mechanisms to cope with stress, expectations, and pressure, gradually binding you in chains far from noticeable but no less dangerous.

But fear not, we're here together, and together we'll conquer this veiled enemy. With every word inscribed in this chapter, you're embarking on a journey, leading you from awareness to understanding, from detection to overcoming. Each section of this chapter is carefully created to help you decipher the impact of addiction on mental health, its subtle signs, and the psychological triggers that lead to dependencies.

We'll begin by unraveling the realities of addiction, the degrading dance with dependencies. It's not a journey of mere words; it's an experience, a revelation that will shatter myths and help you see how such dependencies can subtly erode your hard-earned success and mental peace.

Together, we will explore the underlying layers of addiction, exploring the unholy alliance that binds mental health struggles and addiction. We'll navigate through the threads of deceit, educating ourselves about the subtle signs of emerging addiction, a knowledge crucial for early detection.

And the best part? We won't stop at acknowledging the problem; we will stride fearlessly towards solutions. We'll dive into the root causes of addiction, understand psychological triggers, and how to dismantle them. We'll equip ourselves with the knowledge necessary to break free, to decode the psychology of addiction.

As you explore these pages, you'll find yourself envisioning the map of escape, from addiction to liberation. Gain practical, effective strategies and therapeutic interventions catered to high-achievers, enabling you to break free from the chains of dependencies.

Ultimately, the aim is not just freedom, but a rebirth. A reaffirmation of our self, gratitude, appreciation, and a life beyond addiction. By the end of this chapter, you'll hold a triumphant affirmation close to your heart, "I am not a captive to my cravings. I am a master of my mind, resilient in my resolve. Through gratitude and commitment, I break free from addiction, embracing a life of peace, fulfillment, and success."

As we open this riveting chapter on addiction, let us remind ourselves of the principle guiding us through the following sections: "Mastering the mind, we break free from addiction's chains: to know freedom, we first grasp the cage." Remember, freedom isn't a destination; it's a journey. A journey that begins with knowledge, understanding, and self-reflection, leading to effective strategies, resources, and the determination to break free.

Without further ado, let's move straight into understanding and overcoming this concealed enemy, holding hands with determination, courage, and an unflinching belief in our ability to reclaim control over our lives. The high-powered lifestyle can be demanding, but guess what? You're stronger. You're resilient. And yes, you can break free.

Let's dive in, shall we?

The Degrading Dance with Dependency: An Intimate Encounter with the Shadows of Success

There's an uncanny allure to the constellation of success, a magnetism that draws us towards its radiant glow, promising satisfaction, fulfillment, and the dazzling badge of societal validation. As high achievers, you've chased this glistening beacon, propelled by audacious ambition, unyielding determination, and an unwavering belief in your potential. Yet beneath the glow of success, under the brilliant constellation, lurks a clandestine adversary – the dance with dependency.

Yes, addiction sears into the core of high-power environments and success-driven lifestyles, enticing individuals into its deceptively comforting rhythm. As masked participants in this dance, individuals might find temporary solace in its deceptive harmony amidst the professional pressures, the relentless stress, and mounting expectations. It sneaks in under the harmless guise of a coping mechanism, blurring the line between habit and dependency until it choreographs your life.

The echoing whispers of a high-paced lifestyle darken the stage, each demand, each challenge, a resonant beat in the symphony of addiction. As high-achievers, your professional commitments might propel you into rhythmically intertwined patterns of stress management and coping mechanisms, paving the way to dependency. But what does this dependency, this dance with the shadows, entail?

Dependency – it seizes control subtly, infiltrating daily routines and intricately woven into the fabric of your life's rhythm. It could be a socially acceptable glass of wine after a grueling day, a seemingly harmless candy bar consumed amidst an engrossing project, or the unending cycle of overwork that blurs the lines between professional commitment and unhealthy obsession. What begins as an occasional indulgence or a coping technique gradually morphs into a relentless dependence, silently dictating your life's movements.

Intertwined in this dance with dependency are the precarious dimensions of mental health. The challenges you weather, the stress you shoulder, they don't just leave a tangible impact on your professional life and personal relations, but they also stir waves in the delicate ocean of your mental health. The power-packed pressure of maintaining professional excellence and fulfilling personal responsibilities can provoke anxiety, amplify stress, and heighten susceptibility to addiction.

Imagine your life, your journey, as an intricately painted landscape across a vast canvas. Threads of joy, splashes of triumph, stains of setbacks, smudges of challenges – each streak forming the vibrant story of your journey. But imagine a dense, black fog sneaking in, consuming the colors, diluting the intricate design. That fog – the insidious haze of dependency – can dim your victories' glow, obscure the clarity of your dreams, and taint your relationships' essence.

However, recognizing this dance, acknowledging the rhythm of dependency, is the first step to reclaiming the artistry of your life canvas, refining the strokes tainted by addiction. Recognize that you're more than your professional achievements, that your worth extends beyond societal validation, outside your contribution to the client's project, or sterling performance in board meetings.

The understanding goes deeper than recognizing the evident signs of addiction; it's a heart-to-heart with your soul, peeling back the layers of social conditioning and societal expectations, and unraveling the naked truth. However, this truth, while momentarily daunting, is empowering, and liberating.

As you journey through this exploration, you'll realize that the dance with dependency doesn't dictate your worth or your life's rhythm. It's a temporary stumble, a momentary misstep. And remember, every misstep is an opportunity to correct your stance, refine your movements, and dance again – this time, to the rhythm of resilience, freedom, and authentic happiness.

Let's journey further into the unholy alliance between mental health struggles and addiction, intertwined threads in the tapestry of high-power lifestyles. Let's pledge to navigate this exploration with courage, reminding ourselves of our inherent resilience while unmasking the silent predator. Let's stride confidently toward understanding, acceptance, and ultimate liberation. Together, we've got this.

The Dark Duo: Tracing the Sinister Alliance Between Mental Health and Addiction

The dance with dependency, although disguised as a deceptive harmony amidst an ambitious, success-driven lifestyle, doesn't tango solo. In the complex choreography of high-powered living, this deceptive dance forms an unholy alliance with a formidable partner – mental health struggles.

Picture the high-power environment as a storm-swept sea, where each demanding wave threatens to destabilize the boat of your mental equilibrium. The noisy cacophony of stress, pressure, success-chasing, societal expectations, and personal battles roar in unison like an unforgiving tempest. The lone vessel in the tumultuous waters is your mind, attempting to stay buoyant amidst the maelstrom. The vessel's strength and stability lie in your mental health, its integrity compromised by these ceaseless waves.

Our understanding journey now wades into the murky waters of the link between addiction and mental health - a connection intertwined with the fabric of high-achieving lifestyles. This duo dances hand in hand under the glimmering chandeliers of corporate offices, within the confined corners of our homes, amidst the hustle and bustle of city life, and in the quiet solace of solitude.

Mental health challenges such as burnout, anxiety, depression and sleep disorders, often twirl on the dance floor, as partners to addiction problems. The relentless pressure of maintaining professional excellence and fulfilling personal responsibilities can lead to anxiety, which in turn may develop dependency habits as a means of escape.

Take, for example, Jack. An exemplary leader, admired at the office for his relentless drive and impeccable work. Yet, unbeknownst to his peers, he grapples with overwhelming anxiety and the constant nagging itch of self-doubt. He's found his partner in the dance – a bottle of whiskey conveniently tucked away in the corner office. With each glass consumed, his fears temporarily hush, the pressures recede, and he feels invincible. The nocturnal silence of his home echoes the whispers of dependency, an insidious choreographer, guiding him in its dance.

Similarly, Lily, a top-tier executive and a loving wife, shoulders the mantle of excellence both at home and in the corporate arena. The increasing stress leads to depressive spells, inviting an unfamiliar partner into her life, a habit of emotional eating. The comforting clasp of unhealthy food veils her pain temporarily, but silently chains her in its rhythm, orchestrating a dangerous dance.

It's crucial to acknowledge that this alliance between mental health struggles and addiction intensifies the throbbing pain of the struggle. It erodes the barriers of mental resilience, induces detrimental dependency patterns, engenders self-doubt, and dims the beacon of self-love. But the dance isn't over. The music hasn't stopped. As vital as it is to acknowledge the dangerous duo, it is equally essential to believe that this choreography can change, the rhythm can shift, and the dancers can chart a new course.

Let's not allow this unholy alliance to define our value or orchestrate our lives. We contain multitudes beyond societal validation and professional achievement. In the journey towards understanding, accepting, and ultimately liberating ourselves from the chains of addiction, let's be guided not by the rhythm of our struggles, but by the melody of our resilience.

As we molt our fears and liberate ourselves from this unhinged dance, let's remember that self-acknowledgement is not an admission of defeat. It's the first step towards victory, toward liberation, and towards self-empowerment.

Let's further understand these disguised dancers. Let's move ahead, to recognize the subtle signs of an emerging addiction that even the vigilant ones can miss. To know how it cloaks itself as a harmless habit before ruthlessly dictating your life's movements. Suits on, masks off, hurdles ahead, but with courage in our hearts and determination in our spirits, we've got this. Let us strive together toward a life of resilience, freedom, and authentic happiness. Together, we're unstoppable.

Unveiling the Mask: Deciphering the Subtle Signs of Growing Addiction

As we continue our journey through understanding and overcoming the dependencies plaguing high-powered lifestyles, we now arrive at a crucial stage. The quiet, insidious onset of addiction can often sneak past even the most vigilant of us, cloaked in the guise of harmless habits and seeming innocuity, continuously pulling the strings from behind the scenes. However, once spotlighted and acknowledged, this camouflage begins to unravel, and the facade of the charade comes tumbling down.

The sneaky subtleties of addiction are often seen through changes in behavior, appearance, health, and even relationships. This ticking time bomb might masquerade itself as frequent forgetfulness, chronic insomnia, uncharacteristic paranoia or inability to focus, gradually etching a deeper and darker presence into your life.

Subtle alterations in your daily routine, which you may dismiss as stress-induced or transient, could be red flags signaling an imminent danger. It's like an unwelcome guest, quietly tiptoeing into the grand party of your life, hushing conversations, dimming the lights, and subtly changing the music's rhythm, making everyone dance to its sinister beat.

Let's revisit Jack, our protagonist from the previous section. There were signs, the achingly empty whiskey bottles hidden in his office cabinet, the tired eyes that masked a sleepless night, the shaky hands during the board meeting, the increasing isolation, and the sudden, almost drastic weight loss. All were unassuming signs of the silent predator lurking in the shadows, pushing him deeper into its pulsating rhythm.

Similarly, Lily's habitual overindulgence in food, her withdrawal from social circles, her dawning emotional volatility, and her unaccounted bouts of sadness were warning signals, faded sirens whispering the advent of the deceiving dance of addiction.

Recognizing these subtle signs is an empowering tool in our journey towards understanding and dominance over our dependencies. Once identified, they become significant milestones guiding us away from the deviant path that addiction lays out, pushing us forward towards liberation and resilience.

The shift towards a balanced, fulfilling, and dependency-free existence requires courage and readiness to recognize and understand these signs. They will serve as stepping stones, paving the way towards decoding the complex web of addiction, and ultimately breaking free from its clutches.

As we unearth the subtle whispers of emerging addiction, let's embark on a more profound journey – decoding the psychology of addiction. Let's understand the roots, peeling back the layers of the mysterious onion that is addiction. Let's venture into the unseen realms of psychological triggers and interpersonal factors that invite addiction to settle into our lives.

Competing with dependency is not a sprint; it's a marathon. It's about enduring, standing tall in face of adversity, facing our challenges head-on, and being brave, even when the odds are against us. It's not about the speed; it's about the resilience, one step at a time, one day at a time. It calls for courage but remember, we are together on this journey. Hand in hand, we walk toward resilience, freedom, and authentic happiness. Let's keep walking.

The Tangled Underbelly: Decoding the Psychology of Addiction

The journey thus far has enlightened us about the hide-and-seek game addiction plays with our lives. We've drawn back the veil, exposing the subtle signs that may point to an emerging addiction. Now, we dive deeper, into the shadowy labyrinth beneath the surface - the psychology of addiction.

The roots of our dependencies burrow deep into the varied soils of our personal experiences, genetic predispositions, social environments, and even, ironically, our accomplishments and victories. Our understanding of these roots is a lynchpin in breaking free from the chains of addiction.

Imagine addiction as an invasive weed, creeping silently into the garden of your mind, drawing strength from factors such as high stress levels, past traumas, or neurobiological anomalies. The weed sprouts, unnoticed in the lushness of your garden, encouraged by societal pressures and psychological vulnerabilities that high achievers often face.

Remember Jack's predicament? Behind the scenes of his success was an unhealthy association, linking relaxation and temporary respite from anxiety with the consumption of alcohol. Lily, on the other hand, found comfort from stress and a false sense of control in overeating. Without realizing, both allowed these dependencies to dictate their coping mechanisms, gradually giving rise to addiction.

Our emotional and psychological reactivities significantly contribute to the development and perpetuation of addiction. Regrettably, in high-stakes professional settings, mental resilience sometimes buckles under the weight of expectations, paving the way for addiction.

Yet, understanding the psychological underpinnings of addiction isn't about imposing blame on oneself, but about facilitating the path toward resilience and liberation. It's about using this understanding as a compass, pointing us towards the strategies and coping mechanisms required to break free from the sinister dance of addiction.

As we peel back the layers, revealing the vulnerable underbelly of our addictions, let's bear in mind that we are not our past or our mistakes. They're mere chapters in our life's colorful anthology, not the entire story. Let's rewrite the narrative. Let's write a story of strength, resilience, and liberation.

Now that we've decoded the depths of our dependencies, we're equipped with the knowledge, the empathy, and the courage to confront them head-on. We're ready to chart our path out of the gloom, towards the dawning horizon of liberation. In our pursuit of a wholesome, fulfilled, and addiction-free life, to liberate ourselves doesn't entail only the breaking of chains; it involves crafting a purpose-driven, balanced lifestyle that reinforces mental fortitude and personal fulfillment.

As we step forward, it's essential to remember that we're not alone on this journey. Together, we'll map our escape route, leveraging practical strategies, therapeutic interventions, cognitive reprogramming, and our inherent resilience to break the chains of addiction and seize control of our narrative.

Girded with self-belief, resilience, and the envisioned purpose of a life beyond addiction, let us stride forward, leaving the shadows behind. Understanding the psychology of our addiction is not the end, but a potent beginning. It's the empowering prelude to the exhilarating opera of liberation, self-love, and a lifetime of authentic happiness. Let's embrace the upcoming chapters of freedom and recovery in our journey, for together, we are resilient. Yes, together, we are unstoppable.

Charting the Path: From Addiction to Liberation

In the course of our unfolding journey, we've journeyed through the dark alleyways of addiction, walked past the subtle signs, and have now unraveled its deeply entrenched roots. Conscious of the psychological underpinnings that may potentially stumble us into its arms, we stand at a critical juncture, prepared to map our route toward liberation, ready to seize control in our narrative.

Wielding our knowledge about our past mistakes and vulnerabilities and our understanding of addiction's mind game, we are equipped to strategize our escape. Together, we'll embark on this mission, for we are not just survivalists, but adventurers steering our lives towards uncharted territories of happiness and fulfillment.

Grasping firmly onto the tenets of assertiveness, we learn to confidently express our rights and desires without inhibiting others from expressing theirs. Imagine standing firm during a boardroom debate, not backing down on your views yet respectfully acknowledging the perspectives of your colleagues, channeling this assertive spirit into refusing addictive impulses.

The journey of liberation also calls for structured routines grounded in consistency and predictability. These routines serve as beacons, guiding us through the unpredictable sea of stress, uncertainties, and triggers. Incorporating healthy dietary habits, regular physical exercise, and ample sleep into our daily agenda lays the foundation to build mental resilience and fortitude.

The vessel that carries us towards liberation isn't armored with only personal strategies. Professional help in the form of therapists or psychiatrists plays a pivotal role in our redemption saga. Therapy can serve as a rejuvenating oasis, nurturing self-esteem, fostering emotional regulation, and effectively confronting episodes of relapse.

Furthermore, mindfulness and meditation lead us to the tranquil shores of mental fortitude and resilience. Witnessing our thoughts and emotions without judgment, we gain the ability to respond instead of impulsively reacting to stressors and triggers. We learn to embrace the calm within the storm, confronting cravings with a composed demeanor.

The addiction almanac also emphasizes the power of social spheres in our liberation journey. A supportive network of friends, mentors, or support groups anchors us amidst turbulent waters, offering understanding, encouragement, and constructive feedback, all while destigmatizing the journey of recovery.

Remember that liberation does not entail mere separation from our addiction. It's about filling the void that dependency leaves behind with enriching activities and interests. Discovering a new hobby, setting personal goals, nurturing relationships, and unfolding our spiritual wings, these pursuits fuel our drive towards a balanced, holistic lifestyle.

We must remember that each step we take, irrespective of its size, is a testament to our indomitable spirit and resilience. Every decision to reject addictive stimuli, every insight we gain about our triggers, each day that passes in the quest of our better selves, is a victory. Celebrate these wins, for they bolster our strength and reinforce our belief in our capacity to steer clear of dependencies.

The journey towards liberation isn't devoid of bumps. There will be days of testing determination, of severe cravings, of past shadows looming large. But with each wave we brave, we grow resilient, we grow stronger, and we learn to sail smoother. Lean on this awareness as we advance, for the road ahead is a testament to our victory over the past and a beacon of hope for a future driven by freedom, mental vigor, and resilience.

As we seal this segment of our journey, let's not forget that our liberation is more than just breaking free; it's about soaring above, about rediscovering our strengths, reclaiming our narrative. Liberation is the dawn of rebirth and marks the beginning of a lifelong commitment towards maintaining this newfound freedom. It paves the way towards gratitude, appreciation and a life unshackled, fostering the self-belief, "I am not a captive to my cravings. I am a master of my mind, resilient in my resolve. I am ready to embrace a life beyond dependency."

Together, let's set sail into this horizon, towards an empowering life beyond addiction, and in the process, establishing peace, fulfillment, success, and authentic happiness as our new norm. Let's continue to keep marching forward, for together, we are resilient. Yes, together, we are unstoppable.

The Triumph: Gratitude, Appreciation, and Life Beyond Addiction

Emerging from the labyrinth of addiction, we stand at the threshold of a grand and magnificent journey where we meet our true selves, where we realize our indomitable spirit. Now, poised at this critical juncture, prepared to launch our lives toward the fascinating territories of happiness and fulfillment, it's time we acknowledge what we've conquered and express gratitude for our journey, appreciating life beyond addiction.

Our voyage thus far has lent us invaluable insights, pushing us past our fears and doubts, unmasking our vulnerabilities. It's time to honor ourselves – the mere act of journeying through these struggles is commendable. Even before we are relieved of our chains, the very resolve to conquer our addiction is victory in itself. It's our resilient spirit manifesting itself.

Each chapter in our journey, each test of resilience, each breaking point that we've overcome, has appended to our strength, has fortified our will. This journey has unraveled our true self – a self where determination pierces through the fog of addiction, where resolve trumps fear. A self that appreciates life's contrast, gleaning lessons from trials and tribulations.

Embracing gratitude is a transformative resolution. It shifts our focus from what's missing, to what's there. We begin acknowledging the strength that propelled us past our struggles and we start to value the individuals who stood by us, lending their support and comfort when we most needed it. Our perspective starts to shift as we orient towards positive emotions, relishing personal victories and joyous moments.

Now, as we venture into a life beyond addiction, we're not merely renouncing an old habit. We commit to birthing an enriched version of ourselves – a person who radiates resilience, confronts vulnerabilities, and embodies a spirit of relentless pursuit of self-improvement.

To maintain our newfound freedom, we need to create a fulfilling life that offers more than what the addictive substances or behaviors used to provide. Designing a life that engages and gratifies us can prevent relapses while also fostering a sense of achievement.

Our journey doesn't end here. This path of self-discovery, personal growth, and liberation, is a continuous one. The resilience and courage we've shown thus far must be harnessed as we strive for greater aspirations beyond our dependencies. We vehemently define our identity, tracing a trajectory branching out from where we stand today – triumphant, liberated, and illuminated.

As we wind down this chapter, let's hold onto the affirmation:

"I am not a captive to my cravings. I am a master of my mind, resilient in my resolve. Through gratitude and commitment, I break free from addiction, embracing a life of peace, fulfillment, and success."

Let this creed guide us, cementing our path forward, reminding us of our capability in carving our destiny.

In the quiet spaces of our heart, let's applaud our journey, rejoice our transformation, celebrate the awakened and enlightened "me." Let's hoist our sails high, ready to venture into uncharted waters of self-understanding, self-esteem, empowering insights, and unprecedented growth.

Welcoming an era of thriving beyond addiction, let's embark on our next journey, the journey to redefine our perspective, where we deliberate on our identity and self-esteem in high-powered lifestyles. Here, we continue our voyage, recognizing our true selves, celebrating our worth, and forging a stronger, resilient, and vibrant identity. Yes, together, we are resilient. Yes, together, we are unstoppable.

5

Self-Perspective Playbook: A Practical Guide to Reconceiving Identity and Self-esteem in High-Powered Leaders

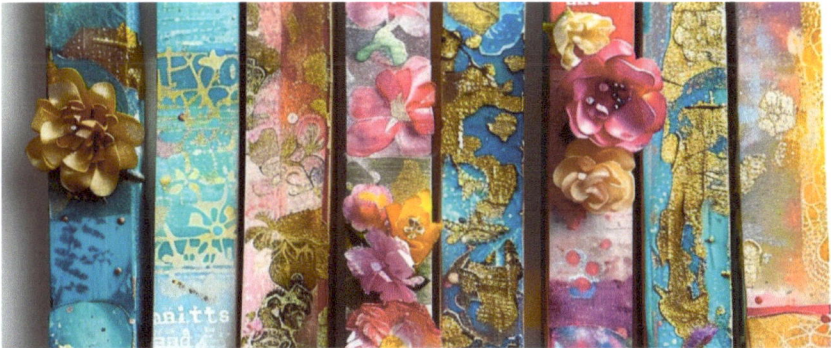

To master leadership, one must first master self - in truth, acceptance, and valiant self-affirmation, lies the conquering of self-doubt.

Welcome, high-achievers, leaders in your field, crafting success stories that are the stuff of envy but wrestling with the invisible battles within. This chapter, 'Self-Perspective Playbook: A Practical Guide to Reconceiving Identity and Self-esteem in High-Powered Leaders,' is not just another chapter. It is an empowering voyage of self-discovery, a rallying call for you to decode your self-perception, unravel the layers of your identity, and confront the lurking self-doubt.

Through these pages, we'll walk the tightrope strung between your public image and mirror image, between your stirring successes and drowned doubts, between your celebrated achievements and clandestine anxieties. Far too often, the world sees you basking in the glow of external accolades while missing the undercurrent of inner turmoil. But remember, it is 'you,' the true 'you' that matters, not the version curated for the world's view.

In the realm of leadership, the journey commences from within. Honing leadership skills or wielding influence isn't merely about mastering the art of negotiation, strategic planning, or effective communication. At its core, it's about mastering yourself. For, in the dance of leadership, you cannot truly lead others until you've learned how to lead yourself.

The driving principle that we address ensures we keep our focus on the reflection in the mirror. Before we journey to the outer world's farthest corners, we need to embark on the journey within. To master leadership, one must first master self - in truth, acceptance, and valiant self-affirmation, lies the conquering of self-doubt.

Let's navigate these pages together, not as relentless high-achievers or influential leaders but as fellow humans with dreams, doubts, strengths, and fears. Let's learn to differentiate between the face in the mirror and the mask we occasionally wear. Let's closely examine the influence of self-image on our lives and perceive the dance of constant paradox between public success and private self-doubt.

This chapter will help you understand that you are not alone in dealing with these internal battles. It will enlighten you with wisdom to embrace a new perspective, recognize your inherent worth, and relinquish the anchors of self-doubt that weigh you down. It offers actionable insights to help build a resilient self-image, one that is immune to the damaging effects of comparison and societal pressure.

As we embark on this journey together, remember, the journey to self-understanding isn't just about uncovering the darkness within— it's also about discovering and amplifying the light. Herein lies your promise for this chapter—you will learn to see yourself clearly, accept yourself wholeheartedly, and redefine your success on your terms.

Are you ready to embrace your truth, accept yourself as you are, and valiantly affirm your worth? Then, let's turn the page, proverbially and literally. Let's commence each section, each step of this journey, with a spirit of fearless exploration and open-hearted learning. In doing so, we embolden ourselves to meet our reflection in the mirror, look straight into its eyes, embrace it for all its worth, and say, "I am enough."

As we go deeper into the subsequent sections, let's remind ourselves —our journey isn't about becoming something new. It's about coming home to who we truly are. We are not changing but becoming—becoming more of ourselves.

Every unfolding section in this chapter supplements this core narrative, offering practical wisdom and tools that are your keys to unlock this transformative journey within. As we transition to the next section, remember: the road to self-reconnection and acceptance begins with an honest encounter with you behind the façade. Let's embark on this journey of discovering 'you'.

Behind the Facade: Deconstructing the Constructed Self

Imagine yourself as a well-crafted and intricately designed house. The facade is awe-inspiring, and crafted with precision and sophistication. The world stands in admiration of this imposing structure, blissfully unaware of the hollowness within. This hidden hollowness represents the conflict between your externally projected self and your internal reality - a conflict aptly symbolized by the disparity between a house's exterior resemblance and its unadorned interior.

As high-achievers and leaders, you have grown accustomed to presenting a meticulously constructed self to the world. This facade, shaped by societal expectations, professional demands, personal fears, and self-imposed pressures, shields your true self from the world's scrutiny. Underneath this meticulously erected mask lurks an entirely different persona - the raw, unedited, and authentic 'you'. And here lies our first task— we'll attempt to deconstruct this outer facade, allowing the inner reality to breathe and reveal itself.

In your attempt to lead and succeed, you may have donned multiple masks, each serving distinct roles. Some of them represent your professional identity - the CEO, the executive, the high-performer, the innovator. Simultaneously, other masks embody personal roles - the parent, the spouse, the friend, the pillar of strength. Overwhelmed with the weight of these masks, you often feel disconnected, even lost within your own self. Here's what you must remember: these masks aren't your enemies. They are necessary for navigation in the professional and personal world. However, the problem arises when these masks start smothering your individuality when they become so heavily glued to your face that you feel incomplete without them.

It's an unsettling experience to confront the gap between your authentic self and your constructed self. It's like finding a stranger in the mirror, a person you have been living with yet know so little about. This stranger is true 'you', the individual behind the facade of titles and tags, the person who dreams, doubts, laughs, cries, and struggles just like any other human.

Remember, each one of these masks you wear is a part of you, but they don't define you entirely. You are not merely a summation of societal labels and self-imposed identities; you are much more. And, shedding the layers of these constructed selves will guide you closer to who you truly are. The freedom to unveil your true self, to peel off the layers of conditioned responses, learned behaviors, and societal expectations, unveils the authentic you. The you that is frail, resilient, flawed, and perfect in its own imperfections.

This process may feel unsettling, even frightening initially. Standing bare, exposing your vulnerabilities, tears down the defensive walls designed over time. Treading this path certainly needs courage. Yet, the liberation and sense of self-acceptance experienced throughout this process far outweigh the initial discomfort.

Consider this a call to authenticity, a rallying cry to strip off the layers cloaking your true identity, and confront the authentic self that lies beneath these illustrious masks. Not to discard or belittle these masks, but to just understand and appreciate the difference between the roles you perform and the individual you are.

Taking this step opens a new horizon, a chance to look into the mirror and see beyond the veneer, to truly see and recognize 'yourself.' From this point forward, you make a choice to unmask. To shed the protective layers you've meticulously built. To unleash your authentic self. This choice is an act of resilience, a tribute to your self-worth and validation of your unique identity.

With every layer shed, you will stand a little taller, your gait a little firmer, and your gaze a little steadier. You will begin to whisper the truths you've been too afraid to voice aloud, and those whispers will become roars as your confidence surges and your self-image transforms.

Are you ready to embark on this transformative journey? A journey that seeks truth beyond the facade, that nurtures self-acceptance, and that liberates you from the confines of the constructed self. Then let's embark, indeed.

In this next chapter we begin to unravel the duality of self-esteem in high-functioning individuals, our high-achievers. Don't fret, you're not alone in this paradox; together, we'll explore and confront it in detail.

The Battle Within: Unravelling Self-esteem in High Functioning Individuals

On the dazzling stage of life, where spotlights often illuminate the grandeur of your accomplishments, it's easy to overlook the shadows cast behind the curtains. High-functioning individuals, you, often find yourselves embroiled in a silent war: the battle within. This inner conflict is a paradox, baffling even to the most perceptive minds. The dichotomy of towering success externally belied by a creeping self-doubt internally forms the crux of this battle. So, let's unveil its essence and unravel the intricate puzzle that self-esteem presents in high achievers.

To understand this paradox, you must first comprehend that high achievement does not necessarily equate to high self-esteem. You could be steering your Ferrari against the glittering cityscape, having reached the pinnacle of professional success, only to traverse the lonely highways of self-doubt. Achievement and self-esteem, though seemingly intertwined, are not synonymous.

In the relentless pursuit of success, you unknowingly weave threads of external validation into the fabric of your self-esteem. Be it applause, words of praise, trophies, or that coveted corner office - the external shiny badges of honor start defining your worth. Slowly and stealthily, the need for recognition morphs into a dependency, creating a fragile self-esteem contingent upon ongoing success. This 'conditional self-esteem', as we will refer to it, magnifies not only your achievements but also your failures. This distorted magnification can leave you treading the dangerous waters of 'Imposter Syndrome'.

Imposter Syndrome, the gnawing belief that your success is a result of luck or deceit rather than your skills or qualifications, commonly plagues high-achieving individuals. The backstage of your glorious performance is often riddled with anxious dialogues of not being 'good enough' or 'worthy.' Your self-esteem becomes a captive to these voices, crippling your self-confidence, and ironically, it gives birth to an imposter within an achiever.

It's not uncommon, then, to find you standing amidst applause, accolades, and admiration, feeling undeserving and petrified of being 'found out.' It forces you to don even heavier masks, burying your authentic self deeper beneath the facade. This exhaustive rollercoaster ride between towering self-expectations and crippling self-doubts is the reality of the high achiever's self-esteem conundrum.

By now, you may be wondering if this cycle of self-doubt amplification is an inescapable part of the high-achiever's journey. But let me reassure you: as complex as this riddle seems, it's not impossible to solve. In fact, understanding this conflict is the first stride towards a healthier relationship with self-esteem.

Take a moment to acknowledge this paradox within you. Unravel it, understand its intricacies, appreciate its existence, and then gently place it under the microscope of self-awareness. Remember, the goal is not to eliminate self-doubt entirely - for, as we shall see, self-doubt too has its virtues. Instead, our aim is to recalibrate your relationship with self-doubt and restore a balanced self-esteem.

Author and clinical psychologist Meg Jay argues that the twenties are the 'defining decade,' shaping an individual's life trajectory. But I contend that any age, any moment presents an opportunity for redefinition and growth. And the first step towards redefinition is acceptance.

Can you accept yourselves- both the accomplished professional and the doubting individual within? Can you embrace your paradox without allowing it to suffocate you? If you said yes, you've already begun the journey towards resolving the self-esteem paradox.

As we tread further along this path, we will find ourselves ensnared in a subtle but potent trap - the 'comparison trap'. But fear not, for together, we will learn to recognize this trap and escape its clutches, to help you continue evolving your self-perception and nourishing your self-esteem. Together we will venture boldly into striving for a narrative that suits your reality better than the one you've been telling yourself.

The Cost of Comparison: Escaping the Comparison Trap

Captured in the saying, "Comparison is the thief of joy", you're probably already aware of the damaging psychological impact the act of comparison can have on your self-esteem, confidence, and overall happiness. It's a trap you've likely stumbled into more than once, especially in a dog-eat-dog world where everyone is seemingly in a ceaseless race to the top. For you, high achievers who are constantly under the limelight, the comparison trap can sometimes seem sneaky, practically inescapable. It lurks in the background of every accomplishment, every accolade, every praise, slowly sapping the happiness from your victories as you weigh them against others' successes.

Comparison is ironically two-faced, with both conscious and

subconscious implications. Consciously, you compare your achieve-ments with your peers', measuring your worth on an imaginary scale of success. This can lead to feelings of inadequacy and contribute to the fallacious belief of being an 'impostor'. On a subconscious level, com-parison fuels self-doubt and fear, further deepening the chasm between your accomplishments and your self-esteem.

The intriguing part is, in the grand theatre of life, all comparisons are flawed for one simple reason: we are comparing our behind-the-scenes with someone else's highlight reel. No amount of trophies on their mantelpiece or laurels on their cap can reveal the struggles, the failures, the heartbreaks they have conquered. The overnight success you admire is often a sum of countless nights of tireless efforts hidden from the public eye.

Given the detrimental effects of comparison on your mental health and self-esteem, it's crucial to develop strategies to escape this trap. Rest assured, the following lines won't recite the worn-out advice of avoiding comparison completely. That's impractical, even impossible in certain scenarios. We all have our moments of doubting our place in the world and our worth, and that is perfectly normal, even healthy. The goal here isn't to eradicate the desire to compare in totality, but to channel it into more fruitful, self-constructive phenomena.

Powerful solution to this conundrum? Less comparison, more intro-spection. Let's flip the coin and use comparison as a self-awareness tool. How about striving for a 'benchmark of one'? In this unique bench-marking approach, the person you should be striving to surpass is no one else but who you were yesterday.

Admittedly, it's an uphill task to distance yourself from the toxic cycle of comparison, right? But remember, you aren't alone. We are all in this together, locked in a universal struggle of finding ourselves in the grand narrative of life. It's about valuing your journey, your perseverance, your growth journey, and understanding that there's no universal measuring stick for success.

As we now slowly extricate ourselves from the comparison trap, we also need to tackle the consequent narrative it has birthed within us. The narrative that has been shaped by years of judging ourselves based on predetermined standards and benchmarks; the narrative that desperately needs recasting. As we journey forward, let's march towards rewriting the narrative and transforming our self-perceptions, answering the urgent call to redefine success and truly recognize the unique, exceptional individuals we are. Let's undertake this transformation to redefine what success truly means for each one of us. We are now ready to begin carrying this newfound wisdom forward, into the art of transforming our skewed perceptions and redefining our personal crescendo - Success!

Rewriting the Narrative: Transforming Self-Perception, Redefining Success

In the journey of self-discovery and growth, an important stepping stone is the transformation of self-perception. It is this perception of yourselves that crafts your internal narrative, a narrative that has, up until now, been subtly etched by societal norms, expectations, and the inevitability of comparison. It is this narrative that often fuels self-doubt and chips away at your self-esteem. Therefore, rewriting this internal narrative, redefining your perception of self and success becomes paramount to pave the way for holistic personal development.

Transforming self-perception and redefining success begins with unlearning and dismissing the limiting beliefs imposed by society. Success isn't a one-size-fits-all concept, and your accomplishments should not be confined to predefined lines of society's drawing. The tangible tokens of success—whether it's the corner office, the opulent house, or the luxury car—are not sufficient measures of your worth or capability.

Instead, let's reconsider the metrics of success. Perhaps it would serve better to measure success by personal growth, by resilience, by adaptability, by empathy. Perhaps success is better tasted in self-contentment than in applause. Perhaps success is trusting your journey and appreciating your individual pace, rather than scrambling a race against the world.

The art of transforming self-perception is akin to creating a master-piece of your own identity. You, with your unique blend of strengths, weaknesses, experiences, aspirations, constitute an original master-piece, and it is essential to honor and celebrate that uniqueness.

The path to transformation might seem daunting, filled with trials and tribulations. The hardest battle to fight, perhaps, is against the voices in your head telling you that you're not good enough, that you don't measure up to the standards, and your self-worth is entwined with your achievements. But worry not.

A powerful tool to aid you in your journey of rewriting your narrative is Affirmation. Harness the power of positive affirmations and self-talk. Replace the "I am not good enough" with "I am sufficient and capable", replace the "I can never achieve that" with "I will strive and do my best". Amplify these affirmations until they drown the self-doubt.

Another essential practice towards transformative self-perception is Mindfulness. Stay present, acknowledge your feelings without judg-ment, empathize with yourself, and you'll notice the slow dissipation of self-doubt.

As we embark on this transformative journey, remember to cel-ebrate every milestone, big or small. After all, each stumbling block conquered, each leap of faith taken, is a testament to your resilience and courage. As we seek to redefine success, let's recognize that the markers of true success are not limited to outward achievements, but found within the varied aspects of individual growth.

Indeed, the journey of transforming self-perceptions and redefining success will challenge you. It will demand patience, resilience, and bravery. But it is this journey that will lead you towards personal development and fulfillment, banishing self-doubt, and bolstering self-esteem.

On this note, as we imbibed the art of transforming self-perception and redefining success, let us equip ourselves better and march towards our next endeavor – Building Self-esteem and Confidence. Let us stride forward, navigating through the intricacies of fortifying self-esteem and harnessing it as a powerful tool to conquer self-doubt and foster personal growth.

The Self-esteem Fortification: A Practical Approach to Building Self-Esteem and Confidence

The fortification of self-esteem is a necessary endeavor on the journey to living a fulfilling life. For individuals who lead in their respective fields, it's not so much about the accumulation of external successes, but rather about the development of inner growth, self-awareness, and resilience. Building self-esteem and confidence, then, becomes a pivotal pillar in the construction of a more balanced, less stress-induced, and ultimately more satisfying life.

To begin this fortification journey, understand that self-esteem is not a destination, but a continuous process. It isn't a tap to turn on and off but a muscle to be exercised and strengthened. Much like the high-powered leaders you are, prioritize building of this strength just as you would in your professional pursuits.

A powerful tool in this quest for fortified self-esteem is cognitive restructuring. This technique involves challenging negative thought patterns and reframing them into positive affirmations. For instance, instead of thinking, "I made a mistake, I am a failure," reframe it as, "I made a mistake, but I'm learning and continually improving." The goal here is to exercise your agency over your thoughts, thus enabling a healthier and more resilient mental framework.

Next on the journey is the practice of assertiveness. In a world where you're often obliged to compromise for the bigger picture, it's vital to strike a balance. Assertiveness does not mean being arrogant or selfish; it means communicating your needs and setting healthy boundaries. It's about valuing your feelings, ideas, and beliefs and expressing them with respect and integrity.

Central to building self-esteem is also the principle of self-care. In the midst of demanding schedules and countless responsibilities, it is easy to overlook the importance of looking after oneself. Regular exercise, balanced nutrition, and allowing time for relaxation and hobbies are not frivolous luxuries, but necessary elements that contribute to maintaining mental and physical well-being. These practices ground you, recharge your perspective and remind you of your value beyond your accomplishments.

Lastly, practice unconditional self-acceptance. You are more than the sum of your successes or failures. Recognize that you're a human being in a journey of constant learning and growth, and it's OK to falter. Embrace your flaws, for they make you human. Instead of mercilessly criticizing yourself for every step taken wrong, choose to learn, adjust, and move forward.

Cultivating self-esteem and confidence does not promise an absence of difficulties or failure. However, what it does provide is resilience, perspective, and a tenacious spirit capable of standing firm, even in the face of adversity. It's the conscious elevation of your internal worth, which seeps into every aspect of your life, empowering you to lead not just with renewed dynamism, but with an unwavering sense of self-belief.

Newly fortified self-esteem and confidence make you want to know more about self-acceptance and affirmation. Do not underestimate the power of accepting yourself, flaws and all. Unleash the power of affirmation, and manifest the resilience, the self-belief, and all the mental fortitude you've been nurturing in your journey so far. The process of metamorphosis is in full swing, and it's time to witness the beauty of the transformative ascension!

Introspective Triumph: The Power of Self-Acceptance and Affirmation

The transformative journey that you have embarked on is bound to change not only how you perceive yourself but also how you interact with the world around you. Having fortified your self-esteem, let us now embrace the power of self-acceptance and affirmation. These two elements are key to continuously nurturing the garden of your mind and fostering personal growth.

Self-acceptance is a courageous act of recognizing and owning your strengths as well as your weaknesses. It's about acknowledging your humanness, complete with all your flaws and quirks. Rather than pushing them into the corners of your consciousness, bring them into the light. By doing so, these perceived weaknesses no longer hold you hostage but become stepping stones towards more authentic interpersonal relationships and a deeper sense of self.

Affirmation, on the other hand, is the tool that etches positive beliefs into your subconscious, nurturing your garden of self-esteem, and shooing away the weeds of self-doubt and negativity. Positive affirmations act as your personal cheerleaders, challenging limiting beliefs and replacing them with empowering notions.

The presence of self-acceptance and the use of affirmation lead to profound changes within you. When you accept yourself, you relinquish the burden of perfection and the fear of judgement. You radiate authenticity and start attracting people and experiences that align with your values and beliefs.

Allow me to guide you to craft your personal affirmation, one that resonates with your journey and fuels your dreams. Remember, an affirmation is most effective when it is in the present tense, positive, and personal. Here's a vibrant affirmation that embodies the spirit of our journey thus far:

"I am a unique, multifaceted masterpiece. I acknowledge my strengths, embrace my weaknesses, and am constantly evolving. In my journey of perfection, my worth remains steadfast and fierce. I am not defined by others' opinions, but thrive on my beliefs, values, and self-esteem."

Repeat this affirmation daily, in moments of self-doubt, in the face of challenges. Inscribe these words on the canvas of your mind, let them seep into your heart, and watch as they transform your perception of yourself and alter the way you navigate through life.

The journey of self-discovery and self-evolution may be arduous, filled with peaks and valleys. Yet, every step taken, every peak conquered, is a testament to your resilience and courage. Cherish this introspective triumph, for it is not just about reconceiving identity and self-esteem but embracing the power of self-acceptance and affirmation.

Now that we have equipped ourselves with durable self-esteem, a newfound self-perception, and an empowering affirmation, we are ready to venture further into our journey. What is inner peace? As high-powered leaders, balancing outward success with inward tranquility can prove to be an elusive endeavor. We will explore this delicate balance and unlock the wisdom of well-being, to ensure that success does not come at the cost of your mental and emotional health. Let's continue this voyage, carving out a path to holistic well-being, and learning to cultivate inner peace even amidst unyielding success.

6

⚜

The Wisdom of Wellbeing: Cultivating Inner Peace amidst Unyielding Success

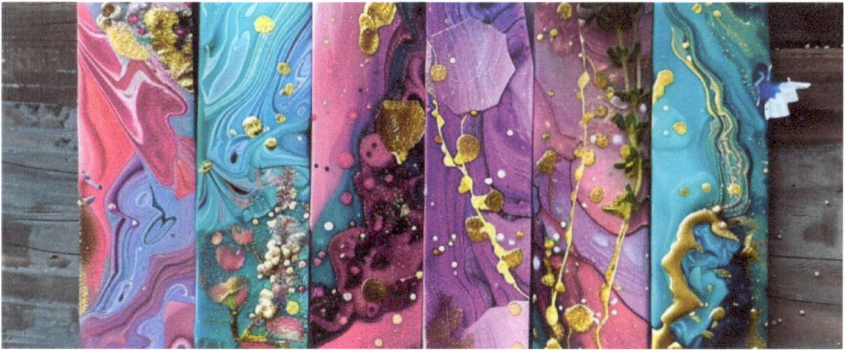

Amidst the tempest of success, cultivate the serene oasis within; for in tranquility, we unearth the harmony of well-being and unyielding achievement.

The journey to the pinnacle of success is often likened to navigating fierce stormy seas. Towering waves of professional challenges, incessant winds of high expectations, and the relentless current of an 'always-on' culture are the companions of high achievers. You, the CEOs, physicians, and executives, often find yourselves in the heart of this storm, steering the ship of your professions while battling invisible storms of stress, anxiety, and mental health struggles beneath the surface.

Yet, success does not have to be a relentless storm. The tempest can be soothed and amidst the gales, a serene oasis of inner peace can flourish. This oasis is not an illusory mirage, but a wellspring of tranquility that sustains, revitalizes, and empowers you beyond your professional achievements. It is this wisdom of well-being that this chapter aims to unfold and imbue in your journey.

Drawing from the principle of this chapter, let's dive into the heart of the storm and, contrary to instinct, not struggle against but soothe it, cultivating inner peace amidst unyielding success. You might wonder, how can calm exist in the midst of such a tempest? How can one remain tranquil while riding the tumultuous waves of success?

This chapter dares to challenge the traditional narrative where high-pressure environments and inner peace run in parallel, never intersecting. Instead, it invites you to conceive inner peace as a critical success factor, a selective strength that enhances, not dampens, your thriving capabilities. Outward success and inner calm, you will discover, are not two ends of a spectrum, but complementary forces that culminate in a life that is not just successful, but also deeply fulfilling and harmonious.

The journey will challenge your perceptions, call you to introspect, provide you with practical strategies, and ultimately inspire you to sow the seeds of tranquility within the arid desert of professional intensity. The chapters ahead offer a wealth of insights, practical strategies, and thoughtful reflections, all designed to guide you in cultivating your serene oasis.

Prepare to unearth the transforming power of serenity amidst stresses, uncover the roots of tranquility, shatter the illusions that have long held you captive, and lay a clear path to inner serenity. Each section is a step towards your oasis, your tranquil hideaway amidst the unyielding pressures of high-profile lifestyles.

The wisdom of well-being offers not an escape from the storm, but an empowering capacity to weather it, to thrive within it, and in due course, transform it. The promise of this chapter is not only equipping you with the tools and strategies to cultivate inner peace amongst success but an affirmation of your innate potential to integrate serenity into your very fabric of being.

As you turn the pages and immerse yourself in the forthcoming sections, keep an open mind and heart. Inner peace is not a distant utopia but a tangible reality that you can experience. Starting from this moment, you will learn not just to dance in the rain, but create a rhythm amidst the storm that resonates with the melody of inner peace. Prepare yourself to embark on this transformative journey, to unearth harmony amidst the tempest of success. One thing is certain: by the end of this chapter, you'll view the storm through a different lens. On that note, let's step into the heart of the tempest.

The Oasis Within the Desert: The Paradox of Inner Peace in a Success-Driven Life

You, the helm holder of multibillion-dollar corporations, high achievers marking new pinnacles in your fields. The world dances to the symphony of your success, yet beneath the melodic crescendo of achievements, resonates a soft yearning, a quiet plea often left unaddressed - the quest for tranquility in the hullabaloo of success.

Could the question -'can calm exist within chaos?'- seem paradoxical? Undeniably, on the surface level, it does. However, delving deeper into the essence of life and success, one uncovers a profound truth. The oasis of calm can and does indeed bloom within the relentless desert of success.

Traditionally, success, with its high-pressure environments and fast-paced rhythm, has been considered antagonistic to the serene spectrum of peace. However, this division is not just artificial but detrimental, discarding a fundamental building block of life and success – Inner Peace.

As the helm holders of success, you are not just achievers but leaders, mentors, and role models. Every decision made, every stride drawn not just scripts your tale but sets a precedent, influencing those looking up to you. Now, what if, with every stride towards achievements, you also pioneered a message of inner peace and wellbeing? Imagine standing tall at the peak of success, the wind of triumph singing praises to your accomplishments. But, unlike the archetype, you also regard and cherish the serenity that breathes within, radiating a reassuring glow of tranquility amidst chaos to those who follow your lead.

Could there perhaps be a more formidable leader, a more resilient success story?

A peaceful mind fuels the dynamo of creative thinking and effective decision-making, augmenting professional competence. It's not the silent retreating corner in the den of success but the vocal fuel powering your cognitive motors and emotional sails.

For too long has inner peace been misunderstood as escapism or ignorance, labeled as a luxury afforded by those detached from reality. It's time to break away from these illusions and reinstate the truth –

inner peace is not the retreat from real-world success; rather, it's the well-rounded embrace of it.

Every tempest of stress faced, every wave of anxiety ridden, and every monsoon of depression weathered, strengthens not just your professional valor but your personal depth as an individual. Inner peace is about being able to face these tempests armed with tranquility. With each professional progression entwined with personal growth, you outline not just the epitome of success but the holistic magnanimity of a human being.

The journey towards uniting the outward success with inward tranquility may appear convoluted, posing challenges often left unspoken in the corporate hallways or entrepreneurial meetups. However, bearing the brunt of these challenges and navigating them not towards avoidance but resilience and illumination, scripts a tale of triumph, gutsier and more inspiring than the conventional narratives of success.

With every stride you take emboldening not just professional prowess but also personal tranquility, you propagate a dual message – being successful and being peaceful are not mutually exclusive, but rather companion narratives.

Residing within your bustling roles and remarkable achievements, there is an oasis of calm humming serenely. This section is your invitation to listen to this humming, to cherish it, to amplify it. And, as you move to the subsequent sections, this humming will grow louder, harmonizing the melody of your success with the rhythm of tranquility. Just as a desert is incomplete without its oasis, may your success story be incomplete without the tranquil harmony of inner peace. On this note, let's continue our journey into the heart of the storm, the storm not of chaos and struggle but one of enlightenment and discovery.

The Wisdom of Wellbeing: Cultivating Inner Peace amidst Unyielding Success

Achievers. Leaders. Trendsetters. You don the crown of success, etching your legacy into the sands of time with every accomplishment. The world commends your exterior glory; however, are you equally cognizant of the interior panorama humming within you? You've mastered the art of dominating the external world – but what about your internal world?

As you sprint the roads to achievement, it's easy, even tempting, to ignore the undertone of anxiety that might creep within. After all, isn't success worth a few sleepless nights, a bit of worry, some stress? Agreed, these might be insignificant costs in the grand scheme of success, but what if they accumulate and slowly, but surely, evolve into a far more unyielding force, sabotaging not just your mental peace but even your tangible achievements?

As high achievers and trailblazers in your fields, you understand the gravity of preventative measures and their role in curtailing the onslaught of unforeseen consequences. This concept extends beyond the purely professional realm and rings true inside your own minds and hearts. Inner peace then assumes the mantle of a skill necessary to prevent the build-up of stress and anxiety, thereby optimizing your mental wellbeing and preventing unnecessary detours on your path to success.

Here's the transformative nugget of wisdom that shall debunk a prevalent misconception about inner peace: It's not a sign of weakness or a luxury reserved for saints or minimalists on the outskirts of civilization. Rather, it's a tool, a strategy that the contemporary, ambitious, high-achiever can utilize to optimize mental health, enhance personal wellbeing, and boost productivity.

The chaos of professional endeavors, financial worries, and personal expectations can brew a heady mental cocktail, often intoxicating your emotional stability. However, this doesn't imply that you're destined for a rocky emotional voyage. In contrast, you can alter your journey by inviting tranquility into your life, by letting yourselves bask in the essence of inner peace.

Cultivating inner peace isn't about eliminating chaos, but learning the art of letting these emotional storms pass without disrupting your inner calm. It's akin to being the mighty oak standing tall amidst howling winds, flexible enough to sway but strong enough not to snap.

This cultivation begins with understanding and acceptance, acknowledging not just your strengths but also your vulnerabilities. It's about making peace with imperfections, dealing with challenges in stride rather than constantly battling them.

The power of serenity in the face of such adversity cannot be overstated. Fueling resilience, positive emotional growth, and fostering deeper connections, it forms the bedrock of your mental and emotional wellbeing, serving a higher purpose than just the absence of discomfort or distress.

Embrace the soft hum of tranquility amidst the thunderous beats of your success-driven life, perceive the reassuring whispers of your mental wellbeing reverberating in your consciousness. Soon, the once burdensome weight of unyielding storms will transform into the bracing winds of change, carving the enigmatic story of not just your exterior success, but most importantly, your interior peace.

As we journey inwards with the forthcoming discussion, bear in mind this pearl of wisdom - Your wellbeing is not contrary to your professional success; instead, they are inextricably linked, one fueling the other. With each step forward, create an echo, an echo resonating the symphony of your success harmonizing with the whispers of your internal calm. And with this resonating thought, let's continue our exploration, uncovering the roots of tranquility and laying our course towards profound inner peace.

The Roots of Tranquility: Laying the Course for Inner Serenity

You've maneuvered the tightrope walk of professional glory and personal wellness. You've uncovered the paradox of how tranquility can co-exist amidst success, and how cultivating this serenity doesn't diminish your accomplishments but rather amplifies them. You've begun to understand that wellbeing is not a luxury, but a necessity, a strategic tool in your arsenal towards holistic success. Armed with this revelation, it's time to commence the next leg of your inward journey, uncovering the roots of tranquility that will anchor you in stormy weather, the roots that will champion your journey towards a harmonious existence.

Manifesting tranquility is a process of nurturing, a journey rather than a destination. It begins with the seeds of self-awareness and acceptance. As high achievers, the process of being constantly in touch with your state of mind might appear daunting, even secondary amid your busy schedules. However, the importance of maintaining this inward connection is paramount. With constant touch comes a better understanding of your emotional landscape, aiding in anticipating and managing the ebb and flow of cognitive tides.

The waves of stress, anxiety, and doubt might feel relentless, but all it takes is the will to ride these waves with grace and presence. Just as a helmsman guides the ship through tumultuous waters with an intimate understanding of the sea, the journey towards tranquility requires understanding and embracing your emotional compass. This aids in navigating the broader contours of your mental landscape, fostering not just success but maintaining an inner equilibrium.

Next, fostering acceptance comes into play. Amid the journey of high achievement, it's easy to slip into the tight grips of perfectionism. While it's commendable to undertake ambitious missions and strive for maximum capability, it's equally important to accept that the road to success won't always be perfectly paved. The pits and bumps, the twists, and the turns - they're all imbued with valuable lessons causing you to evolve. By accepting your path, including its flaws and setbacks, you're ushering in inner peace by embracing the course of life, propelling yourself forward, not despite, but because of the challenges.

Mindfulness, the practice of being fully present and engaged with whatever you're doing at the moment, free from judgment or distraction, is another robust branch supporting your tranquility tree. It's about appreciating the journey more than the destination, the growth more than the victory, the learning more than the achievement. Your moments of triumph will taste sweeter when you savor every step taken, every obstacle surmounted, and every milestone achieved.

Finally, self-compassion and forgiveness form the last vital roots. High achievers often tend to be their own harshest critics. A single failure might result in an emotional spiral, draining you mentally. Here, self-compassion steps in as the balmy salve, allowing you to treat yourself with the same kindness and understanding you'd offer a close friend facing the same situation.

With these roots firmly laid, it's time to nourish the tranquility tree growing within you, lending you the strength to endure storms and thrive in the sunlight alike. As we grow stronger and more tranquil, we desire to understand the misconceptions and myths surrounding inner peace. Let's advance, puncturing illusions and bathing in the profound wisdom of self-acceptance and resilience. Let's continue to turn the pages, flipping through the chapters of growth, resilience, tranquility, and success, journeying deeper into the heart of tranquility.

Breaking the Illusion: Shattering Myths and Misconceptions of Inner Peace

With every step deeper into this self-reflective journey, you've been unbinding layers, recognizing unseen facets, and uncovering truths with each twist and turn. The roots of tranquility, like self-awareness, acceptance, mindfulness, and self-compassion, have shown that peace is not merely the absence of conflict but a consistent, conscious resolution toward equanimity amid success and struggle. As we continue to deepen the understanding of inner peace, it's crucial to strip away the cloak of misconceptions that often befuddle the reality of tranquility and its interplay with success.

Misconception 1: Tranquility equals the absence of problems. It's tempting to think that inner peace comes from a problem-free life. The reality, though? Inner peace is more about your response to problems than their absence. It's about maintaining equanimity even in the face of challenges and relentlessly staying on the course of your chosen path no matter what obstacles you encounter.

Misconception 2: Pursuing Inner Peace is Selfish. Investing time in self-reflection, introspection, or practices cultivating peace like meditation or mindfulness might appear selfish or self-indulgent. However, nurturing inner peace enables you to become more resilient, considerate, and empathetic. By significantly reducing the distractions of anxiety, stress, and confusion, tranquility enables you to become more present, deeply enhancing your engagement and interactions with those around you.

Misconception 3: Tranquility denotes passivity. Inner peace is not about bypassing action or becoming a passive participant in life. Rather, it's about understanding what truly deserves your energy and attention, and what doesn't. It's about defining your journey on your terms and choosing not to get swayed by the maelstrom of distractions or trivialities.

Misconception 4: Inner peace is a "finish line," a final destination. Many envision tranquility as a destination to reach someday. The actuality is, inner peace is a never-ending process, a journey that starts from within and is nurtured daily. Each day offers a new opportunity to add another stroke to the masterpiece of your tranquil existence.

Freeing ourselves from these misconceptions, we begin to appreciate that tranquility is about cultivating a state of harmony. It's about aligning our actions, inactions, responses, and aspirations in tune with our unique rhythm of tranquility.

Having punctured these illusions, it's time to face the journey of embracing inner peace, fostering a mindset bathed in the beauty of tranquil acceptance, resilience. With this newfound clarity, let's embark on the next step, proliferating through the passage of inner peace, inculcating strategies and practices that lace your every day with serenity, ultimately creating your sanctuary of calm amidst the storms of success. Let's continue our expedition, venturing further into the depths of tranquility, surfacing strengthened, enlightened, and revitalized, ready, and excited for the further exploration to come.

The Passage into Peace: An Action Plan to Cultivate Serenity

Having broken free from the illusion of damaging myths and misconceptions and peered deeper into the layers of tranquility, it's time to take actionable steps towards integrating this newfound wisdom of wellbeing into your daily life. It's time to create your personal toolkit for achieving inner peace amidst the unyielding landscape of success.

Action Point 1: Developing Self-Awareness. Being aware of one's thoughts, emotions, and reactions begins with daily practices.

Journaling, meditating, or even taking a few moments of the day to reflect can drastically boost your self-awareness, offering you a better understanding of your internal compass, indicating when you're moving towards tranquility or veering off towards unrest.

Action Point 2: Embrace Mindfulness. Engage fully in every task, whether it's a high-stakes board meeting or a simple conversation with a loved one. By immersing yourself fully in the present, you're choosing to not let past regrets or future fears steal your present peace.

Action Point 3: Practice Self-Compassion. Remember to treat yourself with kindness. Nurturing inner peace involves being gentle with oneself, treating failures not as defining characteristics but as opportunities for growth.

Action Point 4: Cultivate Acceptance. Acceptance doesn't mean resignation. It means recognizing that there will be bumps along the road to success, and that's okay. Accepting doesn't mean we stop working towards our goals. It means we continue seeking growth but do so without an undertone of self-criticism or strife.

Action Point 5: Foster a Mindset of Resilience. Practices such as affirmations, visualization, and reframing negative thought patterns can help build mental resilience. It's about instilling the belief that you're capable of weathering storms, capable of pioneering change, and overcoming challenges.

Action Point 6: Lean on Support. Whether it's a trusted friend, a trained therapist, or a supportive group, having others to lean on fosters a sense of interconnectedness, proving you're not alone on this journey.

The exploration for tranquility starts now, not in some distant, idyllic future. As you infuse these practices into your life, you'll gradually

manifest a resilient tranquility, a stronghold amidst the bustling demands of professional and personal life.

By challenging societal norms, questioning personal misconceptions, and daring to embark on this bold quest for a fulfilled life, a
transformative change occurs. It resonates deeply, affirming the harmony between outward success and inward tranquility. While bringing
down this section's curtain, remember these aren't rigid rules but guiding values. They're akin to instruments in your orchestra of life, each
contributing to the symphony of serenity.

As we prepare to dissolve the section's notes, another stirs. The
time has arrived to examine how this individual melody finds its place
amidst the grand orchestration of life's various successes. Let's journey
together towards the harmonizing symphony taking pride in every
achievement, basking in every note of tranquility, and standing tall
on the magnificent stage of radiant success. Our journey is not over;
rather, we're stepping into the realm of an enriching performance, one
that integrates achievements with inner peace in a dance of harmony
and jubilation.

The Silent Symphony: Harmonizing Success and Serenity

As you've ventured through this enlightening journey, you've navigated storms of self-discovery, faced demons of misconception, and
adopted serenity-rich practices. Now, we are perched on the summit,
overlooking the panorama of your newfound understanding that inner
peace and professional success are not bitter enemies but harmonious
allies. This is the beginning of an unpredictable yet beautiful journey
into the complexities of being a high-achieving individual yearning for
a life that is not just successful but deeply fulfilling and happy.

Having picked up the baton to conduct your silent symphony of
success and serenity, it's crucial to remember that this symphony isn't

played in one go. Just like a musical performance that has varied rhythms, pitches and pauses, this symphony of life is a concert that unfolds through trials, triumphs, and the timeless passage of experiences.

Every self-aware thought, every mindful action, each act of self-compassion, and every challenge accepted and faced leads you to a note of tranquility. Overcome with resilience, every note matters. Every note contributes to your symphony, harmonizing your professional triumphs with inner tranquility.

In the theater of your life, where you've shone brightly under the spotlight of your professional achievements, you're now ready to venture behind the curtain. In the quiet majesty of the backstage, you're orchestrating a symphony of self-fulfillment and happiness beyond your professional glory.

Your mantra resonates, reverberating through the high ceilings of your aspirations:

"From the chaos of my challenges, I rise serene. As melodies of peace resonate within me, my strength is amplified, guiding me to face, not evade, life's orchestras. On the stage of radiant success, I stand unyielding, harmonizing my achievements with my inner calm."

Stand tall, relish in your maturation, your transformation from a dedicated virtuoso to an enlightened conductor that appreciates the importance of mental health, seeks help when needed, and demonstrates to the world that it's okay to yearn for more than just professional success.

Your path to tranquility might have shadows and sunshine, fluctuating like the ombres of twilight. But amidst these shifting shadows and beams, your path is continuously being illuminated. You're steadily molding the concert of your life, and this concert is exquisite for the simple reason that you are both, its maestro and its audience.

In the grand theater of life dotted with flashy performances, your silent symphony can sometimes feel overshadowed. But remember, your symphony is unheard but not unfelt. It can stir hearts, inspire minds, embolden spirits, and above all, it can redefine how success is perceived.

As we wrap up this enlightening journey, one palpable truth remains. The journey to cultivating inner peace amongst the rough terrains of towering success is indeed rewarding. But it's your journey- unique, personal, and deeply transformational.

This voyage towards a tranquil existence amid thriving success does not end here. On the contrary, it gears us up for the next challenging yet intriguing narrative. Prepare yourself as we gear up to redefine the idea of tranquility, exploring its role in our lives, its interplay with our peace, and how it steers us onto paths of unexpected, surprising delights. As we ride this journey together, remember, that you're not just a passenger. You're the driver, the navigator, the architect of the trail that lies ahead. Onwards to the next chapter - the start of yet another thrilling ride!

7

Cultivating a Celebrated
Life: Breaching Barriers to
Unleash Personal Fulfillment
Beyond Professional Success

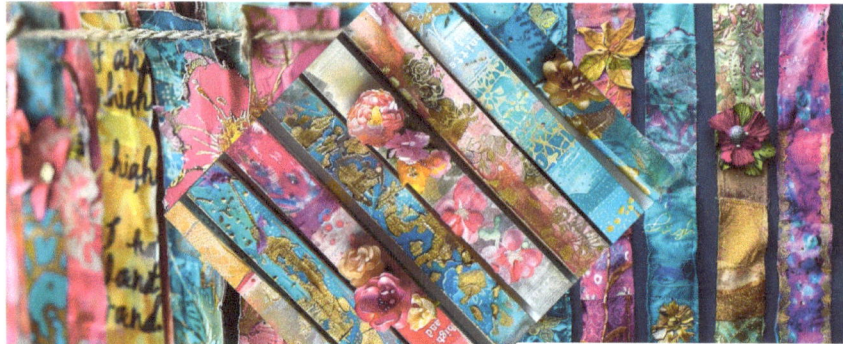

Savor life's symphony. While you mold success, don't forget to
dance to the rhythm of your passion, relationships, and growth.
Celebrate each life-note.

Imagine a passenger on an opulent cruise ship. It boasts all the grandeur you can perceive - glistening chandeliers, exotic cuisines, a captivating view of the limitless expanse of cerulean waters mirroring the azure sky. The passenger is mesmerized by the outward spectacle but silently battles sea-sickness, anxiety, and a sense of isolation beneath the razzmatazz.

The lives of my readers are no different - captains of industry, leading physicians, celebrated CEOs, and executives commanding respect in their vibrant spheres of influence. They personify the grand cruise ship sailing through the mighty ocean of success. Yet, the waves of mental health issues, stress, addiction, and low self-esteem stealthily erode their happiness, marking their life's trajectory with invisible battles.

They are distinguished conquerors, savoring the sweetness of outward victories. But within, they crave a life that's celebrated, not tolerated. This chapter, dear reader, marks our collective journey towards unearthing this desired celebrated life, a life composed of more than your professional achievements.

The harmony of your personal fulfillment, professional endeavors, passions, and relationships create a beautiful symphony that deserves to be savored, not silenced. Each beat in this symphony is a rhythm of your celebrated life - a dance that cherishes every step and sway, not just the grand finale.

Why parade on the world stage with a dazzling, decorated mask, while your soul yearns for unmasked authenticity? Why chase the mirage of materialism, thirsting for joy amid the scorching desert of your concealed discontentment? The odyssey of a celebrated life isn't confined to a linear crusade of professional conquests; instead, it's an intricate dance savored in every twist and turn of existence.

Don't let the chasm between professional endeavors and personal happiness engulf the richness of your reality. Let's strive to strike a melodious balance, a bridge between external success and internal contentment, where neither is sacrificed at the altar of the other.

There's a profound joy that accompanies the pursuit of passion, a peace birthed out of a deep sense of purpose, and a fulfillment that goes beyond just achievement. In deeper waters of your consciousness, you'll perceive your life as a dance, swaying to rhythms of resilience, self-belief, and fearlessness.

In this chapter, you'll embark on a glorious journey, a quest to unlock the door to a life cultivated beyond professional achievements - chasing passions with unquenchable enthusiasm, nurturing relationships with unconditional love, and orchestrating your existence to pour out satisfaction from every facet.

Remember, the ultimate blocks to a fulfilled existence aren't forged externally but within us. Our thoughts, beliefs, fears, and inadequacies often barricade our road to fulfillment. That's why we'll equip ourselves with potent tools fashioned from identifying passions, setting personal goals, achieving work-life harmony, and cultivating mindfulness.

So dear reader, let's embark on this exhilarating journey to tune into the beautiful symphony of a celebrated life that resonates beyond the walls of our professional accolades. In this dance of existence, we are not just the successful maestros but the jubilant dancers, celebrating each note, each rhythm, each beat of our rich, multidimensional existence.

As we step into the following sections of the chapter, let's challenge ourselves to reflect, introspect, and take action. Let's commit to foster a life so intoxicatingly beautiful that we don't merely exist but live, not just survive but thrive, not just succeed but celebrate.

Are you ready to breach every barrier and unleash a life that's not just successful, but also deeply satisfying and happy? If yes, let's stride ahead into the mirage of materialism next.

The Mirage of Materialism: Unmasking the Concealed Void

Dear reader, let's take a closer look at the glinting façade of materialism that often clouds our perception of contentment. It's like standing on the shore of a shimmering lake, mesmerized by its surface sparkle, yet oblivious of the profound depths lurking beneath. The world often tempts us to chase this tantalizing mirage of material comfort, but rather than quenching our thirst, it only accentuates our yearning for something deeper and more fulfilling.

You may find yourself cloaked in designer brands, parked in the driveway of success with your shiny accomplishments, relishing gourmet meals with a silver spoon of influence. You've worked relentlessly to secure your place among the top hierarchy, steering your efficient corporate ship through the turbulent waters of competition. Like many before you, you may perceive that success is adorned with wealth, accolades, and professional prestige.

But let's pause here and ask ourselves - does this sparkling exterior truly satiate our quest for happiness? Or is it just an intricately adorned mask, beneath which our soul yearns for authenticity and a more profound sense of fulfillment?

Don't get me wrong. Professional success, wealth, and recognition are not inherently detrimental. They are commendable achievements, realized through hard work, resilience, and strategic acuity. These are cherished trophies in the game of life, but the game, dear reader, is far more intricate and multidimensional.

Through my years of interacting with high-achieving individuals, like yourself, I've learned a valuable lesson. The luminosity of materialism often conceals a void, a subtle undercurrent of discontentment that often goes unnoticed.

Your professional empire could be expanding, but within, a sense of emptiness may overshadow your celebrations. You may feel like a juggler, constantly trying to balance your professional endeavors with a quest for inner happiness. Unknowingly, we may begin to gauge our worth through the prism of our professional victories and material wealth.

This belief system can lead us into a vicious cycle, trapping us within the confinements of the endlessly glimmering mirage which promises happiness but delivers emptiness. This, in turn, might escalate stress, propel addiction, and inflate self-esteem issues, silently sabotaging our mental health and genuine happiness.

Embracing this reality is the first step towards acknowledging that professional success doesn't necessarily ensure personal fulfillment and internal contentment. When we accept this, we begin to seek deeper waters of existence. We start unmasking the concealed void beneath the mirage of materialism, which is often overlooked due to our preoccupation with outward success.

The thirst for true happiness cannot be quenched by the mirage of materialism. It is found when we dare to look, beyond our accolades, beyond financial prosperity, and nurture our innate passions, relationships, mental health, and personal peace.

Embrace a new dawn of existence, a world where the symphony of success gently harmonizes with the rhythm of personal growth and fulfillment. Awake to the possibility of a life where each day is celebrated with genuine joy, not just tolerated amid the blinding glare of materialism.

In the next segment, we'll explore how to bridge this chasm between professional success and personal happiness. We'll learn to dance on both arenas without losing the balance, ensuring that our exquisite dance of existence never misses a beat. Are you ready to navigate this intriguing journey where professional prowess and personal satisfaction unite to create a fulfilling and celebrated life? If yes, let's gracefully step into the realm of balance - the fulcrum between personal happiness and professional endeavors.

The Chasm and The Bridge: Balancing Personal Happiness and Professional Endeavors

So, you've unveiled the concealed void beneath the glitz of your professional accomplishments. You've realized the need to seek more profound depths of genuine happiness, to beyond the tinted glasses of materialism. Now, let's embark on a quest to find the balance, to straddle the world of professional triumphs and personal fulfillment without tipping over.

The conundrum, dear reader, lies in the balancing act. Tip too far one way, and you're knee-deep in workload, your life a blinding whirl of to-dos and targets. Tilt the other way, and you may find yourself caught in a self-indulgent cycle, disregarding your professional responsibilities.

But let me assure you, this pursuit of balance is not an illusion. It's a challenging but rewarding journey that claims victory not at the summit of success but throughout the climb itself.

So how do we traverse this tightrope? The answer lies in realization and acceptance. Realize that both components – professional success and personal happiness – aren't mutually exclusive but mutually enriching. Accept that balance doesn't mean an equal distribution of time, but rather a harmonious integration of endeavors to yield a fulfilling and celebrated life.

The first step is to set boundaries. While your job requires you to be at the helm, it's crucial to remember that you're also more than your job title. Defining these boundaries shields your personal life from being consumed by professional commitments. It creates a mental space allowing you to switch between roles, from being a career-driven professional to a passionate hobbyist, a doting parent, or a caring friend.

Next, it's about prioritizing. We often jest about the elusive 25th hour in a day. But in truth, life offers enough time for the things which truly matter to us. It's not the shortage of time but the surplus of unfocused direction that keeps us in a perpetual scurry. Identify what brings genuine joy, invest your time there, and watch how it transforms into a realm where personal fulfillment flourishes.

Lastly, cultivate resilience. Sometimes, despite our best efforts, work-life balance can seem an impossibly steep hill to climb. But remember, fellow journeyer, resilience is your compass during such times. It allows us to persist, adapt, and keep journeying towards our goal, despite the seeming challenges.

We now stand on the brink of a pivotal realization - that life isn't a constant pendulum swinging between work and leisure. Instead, it's a dance of harmony, a synergy where these spheres gently sway, touch, mingle, and enrich each other.

As we turn the page, we stride towards a journey that sparkles with the promise of passion, purpose, and deep-seated peace. A journey where professional excellence and personal fulfillment don't vie for dominance, but instead harmonize to create a symphony of success that reverberates within your celebrated existence. It's a new dawn, dear reader, where your life is no longer a juggling act but a joyous, rhythmically-synced dance of balance. Let's gently twirl over to the next melody of our existence, painted with vibrant strokes of passion, raw purpose, and ethereal peace.

The Unveiling of Happiness: Pursuing Passion, Purpose, and Inner Peace

Amid the meticulously choreographed dance of balancing personal happiness with professional endeavors, do you feel the captivating pulse of an innate rhythm? The rhythm of your aspirations, your passions, your essence - the rhythm that leads to the unveiling of profound happiness. In this melody of the transformative journey, we'll learn to not only keep up with the beat of our professional aspirations but also to match the rhythm of our quest for personal gratification and inner peace.

Uncovering deeply seated happiness goes far beyond the thrill of achievements; it's a pursuit of passion, purpose, and peace, all harmoniously interwoven. Passion fuels the fire within, stirs the spirit, and propels us towards dreams concocted in the depths of our hearts. Discovering our passion is like unlocking a treasure chest of joy. It paints our daily canvas with vibrant strokes of satisfaction, making us come alive and creating a life that we truly own, love, and celebrate.

Relishing personal fulfillment also requires an unyielding embrace of our deeper purpose. Our purpose isn't stamped inside our university degree, nor defined by our position in a corporate chart - it's inherent, deeply personal. It's the unique mark that each of us is destined to imprint on this vast canvas of existence. When we align our lives with the compass of our purpose, we set forth on a path marked by satisfaction and a profound sense of meaningfulness. In this sphere, every action, every pursuit, no matter how trivial, becomes a note in the symphony of our celebrated life.

Yet, the quest would be incomplete without peace. Inner peace, often tucked away in the avalanche of pursuits and pressures, waits patiently to be discovered. It's a sanctuary within us, a soothing balm for our restless spirits. It calls us to stillness, to be present in the moment, to cultivate mindfulness. The tranquility of inner peace goes beyond circumstantial happiness; it's an enduring flame that remains unperturbed by the winds of change.

As we journey through this unveiling, it's crucial to remember that passion, purpose, and peace aren't targets to be hit, but trails to tread and landscapes to explore. They don't belong to the destination; they are life-enriching companions that enhance the journey itself. They aren't the ornaments decorating a life of success but are ingrained in the very fabric of a celebrated existence.

The balance we seek and the happiness we yearn for isn't a distant vision anymore. It's blooming right here, right now, within us. Life is no longer a race towards a mirage, but a dance of joy, a symphony of success harmonized with the melody of personal fulfillment.

As we move towards the next part of our journey, let's cognize our accomplishments as part of a broader tableau. A tableau ablaze with professional success, personal passions, a sense of purpose, and ringing with the sweet symphony of inner peace. Let's step into this panoramic landscape where our professional endeavors intermingle with our per-sonal aspirations, brewing a rich concoction of fulfillment that over-flows from our goblet of existence. Let's embark on a new dawn where each day is a celebration of existence, resounding with the echoes of personal satisfaction and professional triumph. Guided by our passion, purpose, and peace, let's embrace a life that is lavishly celebrated, not just passively tolerated.

The Overflowing Goblet: Cultivating Fulfillment
Beyond Achievement

Unfolding happiness beyond professional success, finding passion, purpose, and peace, has led us to this fascinating juncture. We now stand before an unconquered territory, ready to perceive the brilliance of fulfillment that stretches far beyond the horizons of our professional triumphs. We venture into a realm where the accolades of achievement and the glimmers of success converge to fill an overflowing goblet. This is fulfillment not in its limited sense but in its profound magnitude, going beyond our work goals to touch every aspect of our lives.

Consider our lives to be enchanted goblets. These goblets bear every precious drop, representing all the spheres of our lives that contribute towards a fulfilled existence. The professional world is, no doubt, one critical aspect, but it's just one part of this multifaceted goblet of life. A truly celebrated existence sees the goblet brimming over with a rich blend of ingredients. Ingredients such as meaningful relationships, captivating hobbies, philanthropic endeavors, spiritual awakenings, and personal health and fitness, spiced with flavors of adventure, exploration, and learning. This is the fulfillment that percolates into every crevice of our lives, making it truly celebrated and whole.

Visualize the goblet filled to the brim, the elixir of fulfillment leaving a trail of ebullience. An ebullience that manifests in professional success, healthy relationships, philanthropic joy, spiritual contentment, and personal satisfaction. If fulfillment only touched upon the realm of professional success, it would be akin to filling this goblet with only one ingredient. And, would that be a truly satisfying, wholesome potion? Certainly not!

The concept of the overflowing goblet is to challenge you to awaken the facets of your existence that have been dormant. To urge you to illuminate the areas of your life that have been camouflaged in the shadows of professional dominance. To implore that the goblet of your existence is filled with all facets of a rich, varied, and fulfilling life, consistently replenishing it with versatile experiences and learning.

This fulfilling journey is about honoring every part of the life you've built; it's about realizing that your welfare, joy, and satisfaction lie in that equilibrium. It's about acknowledging that your life - your total life - is more than your work, more than your profession. It's about celebrating your existence in its entirety.

As our journey weaves through the terrains of passion, purpose, personal fulfillment, and professional success, it approaches an intersection where each path meets. It's the point where we explore mundane experiences with a newfound curiosity, where shared ventures erupt into laughter, where small wins are cheered as vividly as the big ones, and where every single day is perceived as unique, vibrant, and most importantly, worthy of celebration. Let's move ahead towards that alluring horizon, discovering practical strategies, building blocks of a truly celebrated life. Let's unravel this symphony of a celebrated existence together, piece by piece, note by note, all the while guided by our passion, purpose, and inner peace.

Building Blocks of Fulfillment: Crafting a Life Worth Celebrating

Having embarked on this exhilarating journey of self-discovery and having chosen to be more than just our professional accolades, we now approach the practical steps to further redeem our claim on personal fulfillment. Yes, we've illuminated the concept of a 'celebrated life,' one overflowing with more than just professional success, but how do we construct this reality for ourselves? It's time we dig into the building blocks that help cement a truly fulfilling existence.

One of the first building blocks entails identifying what genuinely fuels your passion, not as an afterthought, but as a deliberate act of self-discovery. This effort helps unearth those enthralling endeavors that captivate our momentous attention and satiate our curious minds. It could be learning a new language, mastering a musical instrument, embarking on photographic trails, or even connecting on a deeper level with friends and family over shared experiences. We forget so often that our hapless hobbies and casual interests have a hidden potential of exponential growth and tremendous pleasure.

Next, is the delicate, yet potent building block of work-life harmony. This isn't about severing ties with our professional pursuits; in contrast, it's about nurturing them while also cherishing personal space. It's about taking a pause and savoring personal satisfaction. It's about ensuring your work fuels your life and not the other way around. Remember, a healthy work-life balance is possible only when personal satisfaction isn't compromised at the altar of professional accomplishment.

Mindfulness, another pillar, when practiced consistently acts as a rock-solid bulwark that keeps the tumultuous waves of stress and anxiety away. It brings forth the idea that the richness of experience lies within the present moment. Let this be a reminder for you to fully embrace the 'now,' to revel in those joyous moments of accomplishment, love, and growth, no matter how big or small.

Don't neglect the value of nourishing relationships. These relationships can act as strong pillars of support, helping you weather any storm. They provide invaluable insights, candid perspectives, bear comforting presence, and ensure that the journey is more worthwhile than the destination.

And then, there are the often-overlooked, yet crucial milestones of physical and mental health. A healthy body fosters a healthy mind, a truth we seldom acknowledge. By incorporating physical fitness—a balanced diet, regular workout, sufficient sleep— we enable our bodies to safeguard our ambitions. Don't forget to prioritize mental health as well, by expressing yourself, seeking help, maintaining positivity and practicing gratitude.

Building a celebrated life is not an overnight task; it requires patience, commitment, conscious efforts, and loads of empathy towards oneself. The path may be uncertain, full of twists and turns, but we're all in this together.

Let's remember, we are our life's master architects and sculptors - shaping it with our choices, building it with our actions, and when required, tearing down old patterns to create a masterpiece of existence.

As we progress further, embracing and celebrating the complexity and beauty of our lives, let's remember that life's beauty lies in its diversity. It's not about just surviving the journey, but thriving in it. Let's look forward now, not with apprehension, but with a sense of excitement, as we dare to sketch an existence that not only echoes professional triumphs but also resonates with the melodic symphony of fulfilled dreams. Let's press on to our next step, reaffirming our commitment to celebrate existence, every triumph, every setback, every ordinary moment. Let's cultivate the exultation of existence and prepare to live a life that resonates not just with professional success, but personal triumph.

Exultation of Existence: Embracing the Symphony of a Celebrated Life.

As we voyage deeper into the perceptive context of truly 'Celebrating Life,' several realizations and affirmations encapsulate us. Breakthrough moments of personal fulfillment are born from our bravado to step out of the confines of routinely professional accomplishments. We have built an audacious basis of fulfillment, one that teems with purpose, passion, connections, wellbeing, and the grace of present moments. We've blended exquisite moments of personal and professional pursuits into a magical elixir of existential celebration. Now, it's time to raise our goblets, brimming with the fruits of fulfillment.

Let's take a pause, reflect and revel in the lyrical dance of our existence. In this moment of reflection, allow yourself to reaffirm one powerful truth:

"I am not just my achievements; I am my passions, my relationships, my growth. I celebrate my existence, every triumph, every setback, every ordinary moment. In this symphony of life, I am not just a successful maestro; I am a jovial dancer, celebrating each note, each rhythm, each beat of my existence."

Embracing this affirmation and imprinting it upon our hearts help permeate the essence of life's celebration into our daily existence. With each note of success you elicit in your professional field, add an accompanying rhythm of personal passion and satisfaction. Draw an artistic swirl with every stroke in your personal life while juggling the demanding canvases of your professional endeavors. Dance to this enchanting symphony, where your professional and personal pursuits, fears, and feats, generate a harmonious flow that uplifts your existence from mere survival to splendid celebration.

Unravel the magic that you've been curating within yourself. Break the shackles and soar high on the wings of fearlessness. Discover that you are capable, valued, and worthy of celebrating life. Believe that fulfillment isn't an external award to achieve but an internal flame that ignites with your passions and purpose, fueling your way to a celebrated existence.

As we come to the end of this chapter, the key takeaway remains: A celebrated life is not a prerogative of a chosen few but an embraceable reality for all those daring to transcend beyond professional accolades. For those willing to unearth the buried passions, who strike a balance between work and personal space, who practice mindfulness, nurture relationships, prioritize wellbeing, and yes, for those who dare to dance to the symphony of life!

As we transition into our next chapter, let's continue this journey with amplified vigor and carry the lessons we've learned so far. Let's look forward to "The Elevator to Elevation: Charting your Path from Stress-Induced Exhaustion to Energized Success," not just with curiosity, but also with a determination to cultivate a life vibrating with success and radiating personal fulfillment. Let's continue to walk the path of celebration, ready to conquer any hurdles and barriers as we chart our pathway to elevation. Everything we've discussed so far has led us to this point, where we explore how to elevate to energized success from the strains of stress. And remember, a celebrated life isn't a destination, it's an ongoing, resplendent rhythm. Keep dancing to it!

8

⚜

The Elevator to Elevation: Charting Your Path from Stress-Induced Exhaustion to Energized Success

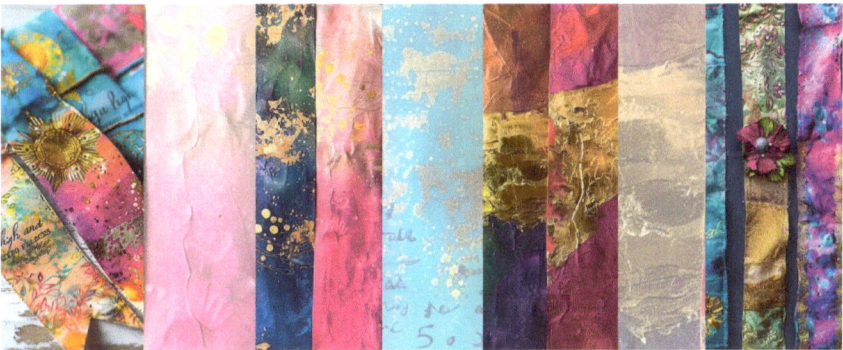

Through capturing the reigns of stress, we ride the elevator from exhaustion to energized success, utilizing life's pressures as stepping stones, not stumbling blocks.

Welcome to this empowering part of our transformative journey where exhaustion does not equate despair but offers an elevator, rising to all-new heights of energized success. Yes, you heard it right! Wave a fond farewell to those days of being encaged within the invisible shackles of chronic stress and fatigue because it's time to ascend beyond. It's time to transform adversity into opportunity, stress into motivation, and exhaustion into fruitful exhilaration! Remember this crucial principle, that we do not just survive our stress, but we conquer it and convert it into a ladder leading us to unimaginable success.

Life, as dynamic and unpredictable as it is, doesn't come without its fair share of stress. In your high-achieving life, where triumph never ceases to follow you, so does stress, unfortunately. The pressure not only to succeed but also outshine, paired with the responsibility to nourish a healthy and happy personal life, often brews a potent cocktail of stress and exhaustion. However, as the influential juggernauts, the unmistakable titans of your respective fields, you've always risen to the occasion. You've turned challenges into trinkets of achievements. And this instance will be no different. We are set to take a magnificent journey from a life plagued with stress-induced exhaustion to an existence brimming with renewed energy, unbounded enthusiasm, and destined success!

Our journey will take us deep within, into the core of chronic stress and its effects, unraveling the invisible yet potent chains it weaves around us. We will dissect and understand burnout, often the unsung villain in our high-performance lives. Armed with this wisdom, we will then charter the ship of resilience, our steadfast companion, to navigate the tumultuous oceans of stress. Coupled with power narratives, essential teachings, and practical tools, this voyage will enable us to rise, braver and stronger, against every challenge life throws at us.

By dispelling the misconceptions about stress, we move closer to appreciating stress as a natural part of life and growth, not just an un-invited imminent disaster. It is detrimental when unchecked but, when appropriately handled, can be our innate motivational force, facilitating us to reach unchartered success.

On this expedition, we are our heroes, reclaiming our lives from stress and exhaustion. Step by step, we will learn to build an unbreakable defense against daily stressors and prevent burnouts. With practical strategies and scientific knowledge at our disposal, we will sculpt our path from stress to resilience, and ultimately, a satisfying, energized life of success.

As we step into the zenith and true essence of this journey, we will learn to unleash our renewed energy, allowing it to redefine our landscape of success and personal fulfillment, beautifully intertwining them as harmonious facets of our lives.

This chapter is your wake-up call, your welcome aboard our elevator from stress-induced exhaustion towards energized success. Let's embark on this transformative odyssey, where pressure and exhaustion become our platforms to ascend to greater heights of personal and professional success. Let's raise these curtains to a life that's celebrated in every aspect and not merely endured! Hold tight as we commence this enlightening experience, as we ascend beyond stress and exhaustion, only left to soar freely and joyfully in our path towards a life that's truly worth celebrating!

Fasten your seatbelts and ready yourself, as we board the elevator to elevation, uncovering promising paths leading from chronic stress to renewed energy and fulfilling success. Remember, the journey is not about battling obstacles; instead, it is about embracing them, learning from them, evolving through them, and, most importantly, celebrating them. So, let's get ready to celebrate this journey of transformation together!

Just as the elevator doors shut, leaving behind ground zero, your journey to exceptional growth, self-believe, and astonishing success starts right here, right now, in this very chapter. Let's ascend, shall we?

The Invisible Handcuffs: Unravelling the Harmful Effects of Chronic Stress

Welcome, celebrated leaders, giants in their respective fields, to an illuminating exploration of a seldom-talked about yet startlingly prominent adversary. We refer to it as chronic stress; I'd like to call it our invisible handcuffs. It's an intensifying force that doesn't discriminate, gripping billions, from successful corporate magnates, renowned physicians to influential executives, in its formidable clutches. You, who are idols for many, constantly radiating an aura of success, are no strangers to this unseen foe either.

Stress is universal, as pervasive as the air we breathe. As we climb the ladder of success, the stress levels ascend with us, often leaving us gasping for breath halfway through. It is an unsolicited byproduct of our triumphant lives. But, while sporadic stress can be a useful motivator, chronic stress, the kind we're dealing with here, has detrimental implications on every facet of our lives.

Elucidating further, let's dissect this behemoth called 'chronic stress.' Just as microscopic germs invisibly compound into devastating diseases, everyday stressors pile up to form what we term 'chronic stress.' Accumulation of day-to-day stress marks the birth of this chronic creature, lurking around, casting damaging shadows on mental serenity, physical health, productivity, and overall life quality. The potent cocktail of trying to outshine professionally, catering to familial responsibilities, and the relentless pursuit to find personal joy fuels chronic stress.

So, how does this invisible foe impact our lives? Ever felt continually fatigued despite getting a good night's sleep? It's a tell-tale sign of chronic stress, sapping away your energy and leaving you feeling perpetually tired. The concentration wavers; even everyday tasks seem overwhelming, and you find yourself caught in the dampening spiral of inexplicable frustration.

Chronic stress, being the deceptive enemy it is, often masquerades as an array of physical symptoms: intermittent headaches, heart palpitations, hindered digestion, sleep disturbances, the list goes on. What might appear as a seemingly physical ailment could very well be a manifestation of stress. It's thereby crucial to listen to our bodies, the silent whistleblowers, exposing the crippling effects of stress we often tend to underestimate.

Ironically, the mental health aspect of stress, despite being significant, is often overshadowed by its physical counterpart. Chronic stress intensifies any underlying mental health issues, amplifying their impact on our lives. It seeds the grounds for anxiety, depression, negatively affects self-esteem, and propels us into a well of self-doubt. It builds a wall, distancing us from connecting with others, including our loved ones, thereby leaving us feeling isolated and undermining our overall life quality.

Stress hijacks our mental tranquility, and if we ignore these invisible handcuffs, we'll unwittingly become prisoners in our minds and bodies. Dwelling within the bustling urban heart, the towering corporate offices working round-the-clock, or away in the serene countryside, chronic stress can silently creep up, unannounced in the lives of everyone.

Understanding the effects of stress, acknowledging its presence, and importance, is your first step towards unlocking the invisible handcuffs. But remember champions, acknowledging stress doesn't imply surrendering to it. Instead, it's about realizing its presence and facing it head-on, ready to combat it! As we move forward, we will explore the many tools you have at your disposal to break free from its grasp. So, let's get ready to break those invisible chains, shall we?

As you turn the pages of your journey, let's further examine the labyrinth of yet another seldom-discussed phenomenon that goes hand in hand with chronic stress—burnout. Let's unveil the layers of this invisible villain and its implications on your successful, yet exasperatingly exhausting lives. Are you ready to defy the trials, spark the desire within, and forge a path to a life truly celebrated? Let's journey onwards, champions, into the world beyond chronic stress!

The Puzzle of Burnout: Identifying and Addressing Exhaustion in High Achievers

Just as the hustle and bustle of a successful life can lead to chronic stress, there's another facet of this journey that remains often unnoticed, hidden under the hustle—a draining, depleting phenomenon known as burnout. Burnout—the word echoes in the halls of corporate offices, the locker rooms of elite athletes, the private lives of celebrated personalities, and the silent corners of your own life.

In its simplest form, burnout is the culmination of chronic workplace stress that hasn't been efficiently managed. A feeling of physical and emotional exhaustion, cynicism and detachment, a sense of ineffectiveness, and lack of accomplishment. The climb to success is arduous, laden with pressure to consistently perform, never falter, and never stop. The nuance being, the higher the rise, the harder the impact of the inevitable fall. As high achievers and path-breakers, you tread the thin line between maximum productivity and burnout daily.

Burnout presents physically, similar to our invisible adversary, chronic stress, in the form of constant fatigue, disrupted sleep, and compromised immunity. However, it also arrives tangled up in feelings of cynicism, detachment, hopeless and a bitter disregard for achievements that once elicited pride. It is insidious, creeping up slowly until you're deep into its pitfalls, finding it nearly impossible to drag yourself out.

You may brush it off, attributing it to an overstretched week or a particularly challenging project, and while it might be so, a disregard for such symptoms could lead you knee-deep into the quicksand of burnout before you realize it. It's important to remember that burnout isn't just a state of physical exhaustion—it's an emotional and mental drain as well. It can lead to a state of work-paralysis, dousing your fiery drive, muffling your motivation, and pushing you further away from your desired goals.

Burnout casts a dark shadow on your professional life; it dampens productivity, creativity, and workplace satisfaction. But it doesn't just stop there. Personal relationships suffer; self-care takes a backseat, and it virtually halts your journey towards personal happiness and fulfillment as well. It's the penthouse view from the towering building of success – breathtaking, yet terrifyingly lonely and exhausting.

Taking an elevator to the penthouse isn't just about enjoying the view up high. It's about the journey, the ride, the exhilaration, as well as the occasional vertigo. By acknowledging the potential for burnout, recognizing the signs, and seeking timely intervention, you prepare yourself to face it head-on. It's about ensuring that the ride to the top doesn't leave you drained at the end.

Realizing that burnout could affect any of us - regardless of our titles, accolades, and achievements - will serve as our guiding light. Recognizing, acknowledging, and understanding burnout is quintessential in our shared journey to lead a life that is not just successful, but also deeply fulfilling and joyful. Because enduring burnout isn't winning.

Winning is learning to balance, to preempt, and to take care, as you navigate the path of driven motivation and unyielding ambition.

Our exploration doesn't end here, for understanding and identifying is only the first step. In the chapters to follow, we will begin unraveling not only the roots of stress and burnout but also unwinding the roadmaps to resilience and recovery. So, let's continue our journey, champions, so you can truly experience a life elevated beyond stress and exhaustion toward energized success!

Resilience Roadmap: Leveraging Inner Strength to Overcome Stress

Now that we've acknowledged the presence of chronic stress and the burnout it can lead to, we are better able to develop strategies for combat and survival. This part of the journey focuses on building resilience, a key factor in the grand equation of personal growth and development. Today, we begin our interaction with an unexpected hero of our tale—resilience, an agent of change, our secret weapon in unraveling the invisible handcuffs of stress and exhaustion, and repainting our lives with colors of joy, fulfillment, and continual success.

Resilience, at its core, is an amalgamation of processes. It's the dynamism that fuels our ability to rebound from adversities and difficulties that life generously showers upon us, especially on unanticipated days. Think of resilience as an invincible shield, a layer of robust fortification that allows you to bounce back not just to your original state, but to a stronger, more holistic version of yourself.

Merely acknowledging the presence of stress and burnout doesn't miraculously alleviate their effects. It's the belief, the fire within you— the resilient spirit—that plays a pivotal role in managing these challenges. Being resilient doesn't imply that you won't experience stress or difficulty, but it helps you navigate through these adversarial tides to emerge victorious. It's your inner strength that helps you adapt to stress and learns to thrive amidst adversity.

High achievers and successful individuals aren't immune to stress, difficulties, or setbacks. In fact, stress and hardships are common plaques on the pathway to success. The distinction lies in the resilience, the adaptability, and the agility that separate champions from the crowd.

Building resilience is like taking an elevator powered by your inner strength—one that lifts you up through overwhelming pressure, stress, and exhaustion. Investing in your resilience is like securing an all-weather insurance, for it stands tall in the face of adversity, radiating hope on cloudy days.

But how exactly do we harness this resilience, you may ask? The first step is to genuinely believe in yourself—your abilities, your strengths, and your potential. It's about understanding that setbacks are a part of the journey to success and not end-points. It's about being kind to yourself when you falter, about giving praise when you triumph, and maintaining a balanced view of situations through realistic optimism.

Let's remember, resilience is not a sprint, but a marathon—endurance and persistence are key. With each adversity you navigate through, each challenge you conquer, you build upon your resilience, molding a more formidable version of you, fortified to face challenges head-on.

As we journey further, we will unearth practical strategies that will help you harness your resilience and empower you to lead lives where stress does not dictate your actions or cloud your judgement. Hold on tight, champions, as we continue this thrilling ride towards building a stronger, more resilient you.

Now that we've started mapping our roadmap towards resilience, let's move forward on the journey by addressing some prevalent misconceptions and mindsets surrounding stress in our next juncture. Let's debunk the myths that continue to cloud our perception and approach towards stress, so we can pave the way to not just a stress-aware, but a stress-empowered life. Onward we go, champions!

The Stress-Free Blueprint: Demystifying Misconceptions and Mindsets Around Stress

The journey towards personal fulfillment and joy, untethered by the heavy chains of stress, requires understanding the true essence of stress and demystifying the clouds of misconceptions obscuring its reality. Today, we explore often deeply-rooted mindsets about stress that may be holding us back and find the means to transform our approach towards it.

The word 'stress' triggers an automatic negative connotation. However, is it potentially not as nefarious as we make it out to be? Is it possible that we have misunderstood stress all along? Let's navigate these treacherous waters — breaking down the misconceptions that confine us and reforming our perspective on stress.

One widespread myth is that all stress is bad. Contrary to popular belief, stress isn't ubiquitously harmful. In fact, there's a form of stress - eustress - that provides the encouragement you need to conquer pivotal moments in life, from public speaking engagements to challenging decision-making instances. It brings about increased alertness, vigor, and an exhilarating adrenaline rush that can push you to new heights. The problem arises not from stress itself but from chronic stress, frequent or prolonged bouts of stress leading to a multitude of health concerns.

Another misconception is to view stress as a sign of weakness or inability. Let's be clear: experiencing stress doesn't mean you're inefficient or incapable. It merely shows that you're human. Remember, even the most successful and high-achieving individuals in the world aren't unaffected by stress. The distinguishing factor is how they manage and respond to their stress.

A prevalent mindset is that stress is inevitable. However, this isn't accurate. You can learn to manage and even harness your stress to drive you towards your goals. You have the power to dictate your response to stressful situations, and with time and practice, you can learn to control your stress rather than let it control you.

Armed with the clarity of these eye-openers, our view on stress is beginning to evolve. No longer are we trapped under smoky veils of misconception, but stand at the precipice of a new dawn—a world where stress can be seen, not as an insurmountable gargantuan but as a tool in our journey of becoming resiliently successful.

In our pursuit of happiness and fulfillment, we have come a long way—from acknowledging our struggles to the resilience that lies within us, to shattering false beliefs. Having debunked the illusions and distortions around stress, our next step is to develop a set of practical tools and strategies. This arsenal will serve as our shield and sword in battling stress and burnout, and more importantly, in drafting our unique stress-defense.

Our journey is not over yet, champions. We've successfully recalibrated our understanding of stress. Now, let us continue on the road to crafting our stress defense. Let's ready ourselves to dive deep into a toolkit designed to minimize stress, eliminate burnouts, and foster resilience. Quite a journey still awaits us, dear champions, as we continue drafting our blueprint to a stress-free, joyful life.

Building your Stress-Defense: Implementing Practical Strategies to Minimize Stress and Prevent Burnouts

The understanding of stress has undoubtedly grown, and the stage is set. We've journeyed through it all - the dark labyrinth of nurturing misconceptions, the blinding fog of stigmatized attitudes, to finally, the breaking dawn of clarified understanding. We are ready now to unleash the power of practical, time-proven tools and strategies that will act as a robust stress-defense system. This next stage holds the keys to an active approach, setting sail on a course designed to drastically minimize and manage stress while also preventing burnouts.

Our resilience, fortified by wisdom and willpower, serves as the foundation of our stress-defense blueprint. An arsenal of practical strategies awaits, aimed at minimizing stress and fostering resilience that gracefully pirouettes with life's twists and turns. These strategies aren't a magic wand delivering overnight results; they demand diligence, practice, and patience to tap into their full power and potential.

The first instrument in our kit is mindfulness, an age-old practice that encourages living in the present moment, emanating a profound understanding and control over thoughts, emotions, and reactions to stress. It helps in taming the rampant stress beast, guiding you to become an observer rather than a victim of life's stressful narratives. The practice of mindful meditation, conscious breathing, and gratitude journaling are stages in this mindfulness journey.

Physical well-being is intrinsically tied to mental well-being, making a well-balanced diet and regular exercise indispensable tools in our stress-defense kit. The benefits of physical activity go beyond weight management - it's a mood-booster, a stress buster, and an energy enhancer. Engaging in a sport, hitting the gym, tried-and-true jog in the park, or even a lively dance session can elevate your mood, releasing endorphins, the body's natural feel-good hormones.

Further down the kit, we find the tool of work-life balance - an element often undermined in our era dominated by hustle culture. Champions, realize that all work and no play, indeed can make one dull! Spend quality time with your loved ones, indulge in leisure activities, hobbies, and ensure adequate rest and sleep. Nurturing personal relationships and hobbies will refresh your perspective and dissipate accumulated stress immensely.

Another infallible tool that we have is professional help. Therapists, psychologists, and psychiatrists are trained professionals who can provide you with personalized mechanisms to cope with stress and other mental health issues. Remember, seeking help is a sign of strength, not weakness.

By integrating these tools into our everyday rituals, we lay the foundation of a fortified stress-management system. This rids us of chronic stress, highlighting a new dawn marked by peace, joy, and a celebrated existence. Our road has been enduring and enlightening, leading us from the thick jungles of burnouts to the greener pastures of stress management.

Now that we're equipped with practical strategies to fend off stress and prevent burnouts, we are ready to take a giant leap forward. Champions, we are nearing the end of this course that charts your path from exhaustion to revitalized success. The zenith of vitality awaits us, where our spirits are immortal, our energy replenished, and our success unwavering. Energy revitalized, spirits renewed — we're ready to bask in the glory of a comprehensive, resounding form of success, teeming with the renewed energy of a stress-free, lively existence. Let's continue, champions, on this elevator to elevation. Let's ascend to the zenith of vitality!

The Zenith of Vitality: Unleashing Success with Recharged Energy and Reduced Stress

Oh, what a journey it has been! We've climbed mountains of misconceptions, dealt with the deluge of doubts, traversed the trenches of trials, and have now, finally, arrived at a vantage point. A point that provides a perspective of not only the road we have traveled but also the path that lies ahead – the Zenith of Vitality. Here, we stand as victors, epitomes of resilience, ready to unleash success from a wellspring of recharged energy and reduced stress.

Pioneers, we have confronted our apprehensions, endeavored to understand the true nature of stress, and sculpted a practical, robust stress-defense blueprint. The captured energy is ebullient, eager to manifest in every sphere of our lives - physical, emotional, professional, and personal. The vigor pulsating within us is now unshackled from the chains of relentless stress and exhaustion. This invigorated spirit, no longer confined, seeks to soar higher than ever.

Rejuvenated and empowered, we are prepared to re-define success, from the narrow corridors of professional achievements to the expansive vista encompassing personal happiness, fulfillment, and mental well-being. Mark our words:

"I am not defined by my stress. I conquer my exhaustion with resilience. My energy is renewed, my spirit revitalized. I am unstoppable, gearing towards uncharted heights of success with each step taken. This is my journey, a journey of less stress, more life, and absolute success."

Bearers of this affirmation, we are ready to reclaim our rightful place in the world. We are the creators of our destiny, the architects of our happiness, and the guardians of our mental health. We are ready to inspire and be inspired, to lead with our weaknesses and strengths, to acknowledge our struggles, and to celebrate our victories.

This Zenith of Vitality holds not an end, but a new beginning to our journey of personal and professional growth. The horizon of success, stretching beyond job titles and bank statements, now encompasses the richness of our mental and emotional spheres. Our hearts, brimming with newfound energy, yearn to meet the rhythm of this vast Symphony of Success.

Pioneers, as we conclude this chapter of our journey, we prepare to embark on yet another voyage. Every chapter, every curveball life throws at us, unfolds into a new awakening, a deeper understanding of ourselves, and our ability to adapt to life's fluctuations. As the curtain draws on this chapter, it lifts for another - one that holds the promise of a harmonious blend of achievements and mental well-being.

The winds of change are blowing, nudging us towards 'The Symphony of Success,' a territory where mental health and success flawlessly harmonize. A realm where our trials resonate with the sound of resilience, where the echoes of our struggles give rise to an anthem of triumph.

And thus, onward we shall stride, exploring this unchartered melody of achievements and mental health. Our voyage across the realm of 'The Symphony of Success' awaits as we continue to orchestrate our journey, each note a rhythm of resilience, each bar a beat of bravery. As we move towards this symphony, let's remember that the melody of life is best played when we are in tune with our minds, hearts, and souls. Let's get ready to be conductors of our Symphony of Success. The baton is in your hands, maestros, play it to your rhythm.

9

Symphony of Success:
Orchestrating a Harmony of
Achievements and Mental
Health

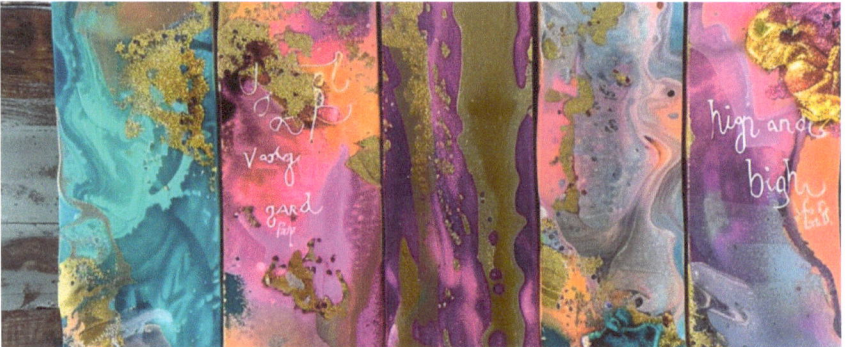

Harmony of mind is the tuning fork for a symphony of success;
balance in internal chords enhances external achievements.

Welcome, highly esteemed reader, to a pivotal chapter in our journey. Smooth pathways to prestigious professional heights have led us to this moment, where we unveil the deepest truths about leading fulfilling lives beyond corporate success. Our guidance is equipped to navigate the tumultuous undercurrents of mental health that frequently accompany the resounding crescendos of professional triumphs. We embark on a transformative expedition to explore the Symphony of Success: Orchestrating a Harmony of Achievements and Mental Health.

The journey to success is not just a solitary march towards the pinnacle but a symphony, a blend of multiple harmonies tuned perfectly to complete a magnificent melody of triumph. The chords of this melody signify various aspects of personal and professional life, with mental health being a constant, dominating harmony – the melody of the mind.

Yet the symphony of success becomes discordant when mental health dims in the shimmering glitter of professional accomplishments. As individuals at the helm of multi-billion dollar corporations or blazing a trail in their respective fields, juggling high-responsibility roles with the demands of parenthood, it is easy to overlook the subtle interplay between professional success and mental health. You'd agree this juxtaposition is often neglected, yet absolutely essential to be acknowledged.

This chapter unravels the principle of a well-tuned mind akin to the tuning fork for the symphony of success. Achievements and mental health are not at either end of the stick; they exist in a continuous symbiotic harmony. This profound balance with the aim of fostering a balanced frame of mind, simultaneously basking in our achieved glories is worth knowing about. Let's jump in.

To our esteemed reader who commands respect and admiration, who is an embodiment of professional successes yet battles invisible mental health issues - our message underscores the desire to live more than just a celebrated life. It advocates for fulfillment, happiness, and a deeper sense of purpose beyond quantifiable accomplishments. The pursuit of mental resilience and perseverance is a fearless journey, a journey we take together.

In these forthcoming sections, we'll venture into profound territories of understanding mental health not as a hierarchical need post-success but as a partner in your symphony, always present, always influential. We'll discover how our minds act as a powerful symphony conductor, keeping the rhythm of our life and success harmonized amidst chaos.

As we move forward, we channel our inner strength, resilience, and tenacity to address mental health issues that coexist with professional wins. This leads us to powerful crescendos of healing, where we highlight techniques synchronized with a high-performing lifestyle, nurturing mental health.

The applause at the final note of our symphony is not an end. It's the beginning of an enchanting encore, a soul-stirring affirmation to continually blend professional victories with mental robustness. The ultimate mantra resonates, "I am the virtuoso in life's concert, proficiently orchestrating instruments of success and mental tranquility."

Let's take a deep breath as we tune up for a performance that touches the core of our great symphony. As we ascend ahead, let's illuminate the symphony's many sections, striking a harmonious balance between success and mental health. So, join us, not just as an audience member, but a co-conductor, in creating this symphony of success - a mindful pathway that enriches the very essence of life and living.

Relish these forthcoming sections with purpose and embrace the transformative journey that awaits. Let the notes of the Symphony of

Success seep in, filling your life with an elevated sense of professional accomplishment and mental well-being.

Melodically, musically, we raise the baton for the next part of our grand harmony... You are the conductor too. Let's journey together towards a Symphony of Success.

The Phenomenal Fugue: Understanding the Ubiquitous Presence of Mental Health

Fearlessness. Resilience. Determination. The journey to professional success often glorifies these traits infallibly. The spotlight gleams on top-tier leadership roles, trailblazing paths, accolades, and multi-billion dollar revenues. Yet, the unsung rhythms pulsating behind these success milestones – the mental health symphony, often lurk in the shadows.

As high-achieving professionals, you have been a virtuoso in crafting an exemplary career symphony, the melody of your success echoing in corporate halls and being revered in your professional circles. But, have you considered the much-needed fugue, the interweaving of an equally essential melody – that of mental health into your life's composition?

Your mind – beautifully intricate, endlessly intriguing, always on a high string – performs around the clock, mastering your professional pursuits, personal relationships, and the constant demands they bring. It often plays the fugue, quietly underlining your career melodies, always present, always influential. Yet, amidst a catena of conference calls, project deadlines, and high-pressure responsibilities, you may forget to acknowledge this phenomenal fugue – the mental health component of your existence.

Remember, professional success is not a one-man orchestra. It's an ensemble with the powerful performer of mental health co-existing and co-operating with every note struck on the success chords. There's a ubiquitous, potent presence of mental health influencing your thoughts, emotions, decisions, actions, and thereby, your success.

Feasibly being at the helm of your professional engagement, high in the hierarchy, also places you at an especially vulnerable place mentally. Which raises an enormously vital question: Are you, in orchestration with your professional success, also tuning into your own mind's fugue? Are you acknowledging the symphony your mind silently conducts, shifting grace notes and stern caesuras, transitional chords, and dynamic changes? Or, are you letting it fade, unacknowledged beneath the dominating melodies of success?

Mental health isn't a hindrance or stumbling stone on your path to success; It's the underlying rhythm, the powerful fugue playing harmoniously and indispensably along your success symphony. Ignoring it won't make the music any stirrer, any more harmonious. It's time to recognize and tune into this fugue – the pressing reality of managing the pressures of your professional roles and personal commitments while handing the often neglected mental health chords.

Mastering this phenomenal fugue, the mental health melody, in symphony with your career crescendos, is not a verse scripted for the faint-hearted. Stand ready for a powerful, symphonic revelation, a score where your mental health deserves its rightful place, its deserved recognition.

Let's clear the misconception, dispel the myth, and resurface the truth – mental health is not an elephant in the room, not a beast to be tamed post your professional accomplishments. It's a partner in your symphony, a critical player, always present, deeply influential, and completely inseparable from your tale of triumphs.

So in our commitment to fearlessly confront the trials, celebrate the victories, I invite you to consciously tune into your mind's melodies. Let's acknowledge and embrace the ubiquitous presence of mental health as a harmonious fugue that, when respected and cared for, can transform your symphony of success into a more enriching, satisfying, and purposeful composition.

Now, prepare to embark on the next phase - exploring multifaceted ways to navigate your mind's melodies alongside your professional crescendos. Like the skilled conductor patiently adjusting their orchestra's rhythm, timbre, and pace, step into the next insightful stage of your journey - examining the intriguing 'Melody of the Mind.' Let's tune into a high-quality performance that not just resonates with success but reflects a well-nurtured mind— fearless, resilient, and triumphant.

The Melody of the Mind: Sailing Smoothly through High-powered Success and Stable Mental Health

Your mind — it's your most trusted advisor, your vigilant guardian, your unwavering cheerleader, and at times, your most formidable challenger. Without a doubt, alongside your ceaselessly thriving professional life, it performs like an adept maestro, leading an internal orchestra, creating the indescribable, intoxicating, infinitely unique harmony that is you.

Imagine your mind as a symphony, playing host to several sections — the strings, the woodwinds, the brass, and the percussion. Each of these symbolic sections has different roles, different rhythms, and different tones — just like the different aspects of your mindset. And amidst the professional ambitions and personal aspirations, there's a section that plays more softly but holds substantial importance - your mental health.

The strings might represent your intellectual capabilities — logic, reasoning, and analytical thinking. The woodwinds could stand for your creative, imaginative potential while the brass signifies your courage, determination, and assertiveness. The percussion embodies your emotional stability, your ability to maintain a steady rhythm amid life's unpredictable tempo changes.

In your mind's orchestra, mental health — it's the understated yet exceedingly poignant fugue, co-existing with the other sections, intricately connected, and powerfully influential. It is not merely a support cast to the leading performance; it creates depth, richness and adds unforeseen dimensions that elevate the whole composition, making it not only pleasing but also memorable.

The tempo of your achievements, the rhythm of your professional success is heartening and well-earned. Yet, how well are you tuning into these aspects of the mind? How proficiently are you orchestrating this grand symphony, this 'melody of the mind,' culminating in a rhythm that not only resonates with success but also echoes personal wellbeing?

Guided by your ambition, you command respect, scaling the unconquerable heights of power. Still, it's important to understand that these commanding notes of professional accomplishment need not overpower the gentle melodies of mental health. The interplay is not jarring; it's harmonious if you know how to orchestrate it aptly.

It's time to become aware – to practice listening to the orchestration of your mind, heightening your awareness to the rhythm and beat of mental health, tuning into its pitch and timbre. This is not just about amplifying your volleys of victories. It's also about deciphering the internal rhythms, the beats that embrace the totality of your mind's symphony.

Learning to listen carefully, you'd realize - the melody of your mind plays the notes of courage, the chords of resilience, and the tune of triumph. Yet, it also hums the tranquilizing fugue of mental wellbeing. Pause, tune in, and begin to value, appreciate, and nourish these subdued, often ignored yet absolutely essential notes.

As you sail smoothly through the waves of high-powered success, remember to immerse yourself too in the soothing waters of mental health. It's about celebrating the climactic crescendos yes, but also dancing to the soft, harmonizing fugue. Let no note go unheard, no rhythm unappreciated, no harmony unsavored in the melody of your mind. You are not the sum of your success alone; you are also the harmony of your mental wellbeing.

In the upcoming exploration, we'll go deeper, confronting the crucibles and celebrating the crescendos as we navigate through the challenging aspects of managing mental health issues amidst celebrated success. Continue this enlightening journey, as we strike the right balance, play the perfect note, and create a rich and fulfilling melody that's uniquely ours. Remember, the harmony of your mental health is not just a part of the tune, it is the tune.

The Crescendo of Challenges: Addressing Mental Health Issues Amidst Celebrated Success

Life can sometimes feel like a symphony being performed in front of an imposing audience. You lead the show, your baton controlling every moment, careening high and low, creating that soul-stirring melody of victories and accomplishments. But at times, the crescendo of challenges emerges, catching you off guard, disrupting your intuitively orchestrated rhythm. Mental health issues, the unexpected notes in your life's score, can often surface amidst your professional zenith, cascading a symphony of uncertainty, a harmony of hurdles.

Stress, anxiety, depression -these are not just words in a medical journal. They are lived realities, often paradoxical for high-achievers like you. The world reveres you for your accomplishments, applauses raining down as you stride up the steps of success. Yet, behind the spotlights, in the solitude of your mind, you wage battles against the invisible forces attempting to muffle your melody. And remember, acknowledging this struggle doesn't take away from your triumphs. Rather, it adds an honest, relatable, incredible depth to your life's sweet-sounding symphony.

Your roles as successful professionals often come laced with an overwhelming sense of pressure. The long, grueling hours, fierce competition, sky-high expectations, striving to fulfill commitments – these aspects do not merely test your skills and determination. They also tug at your mental chords, wear down your emotional resilience, and gradually give birth to anxiety, stress, or burnout. It's a crescendo no one prepares you for. But fret not; confronting these challenges is part of your symphonic journey.

Picture yourself on a stage, each public conquest met with vigorous applause. But each time you bow to take your well-deserved accolades, you feel the unseen weight bowing you further down—the weight of unaddressed mental health concerns. This section is for you to confront and address these concerns, to decipher and navigate through the powerful crescendo of mental health challenges. Learn from the hiccups, move past the pauses, find the strength in the challenging notes, and reclaim your symphony's harmony.

Let's not silence these subtler notes, the hushed whispers of rising mental health concerns. Let's address them, not as signposts of weakness but as markers of our shared human experience. Remember, even in the roller coaster of emotions and experiences, you are not alone—the resonating harmony of successes and challenges echo in every high achiever's journey.

Pause in your pursuit of achievements and tune into the whispers of your mental health. Acknowledge it. Understand it. And when it challenges your rhythm, face it. As you bask in the resounding applause of professional glory, you can also take pride in having faced the crescendo of challenges and emerged stronger than ever.

As we continue our journey, we will gain an understanding of these challenges, exploring how to improve well-being and enhance mental health while elevating success. Finding harmony is oftentimes about having the courage to face the music, learning its intricate notes, patient practice, and embodying its rhythm, rather than merely trying to control it. So, let's explore practical steps, discover therapeutic techniques, and rewrite the score of health in resonance with our thriving professional life. Let's navigate through the music of mental health, one note at a time.

The Healing Harmony: Enhancing Mental Health while Elevating Success

Striking a chord between success and mental health often swings between the battle of harmonizing two complex melodies and finding the resonating note between the two. But fret not, for amidst this captivating musical metaphor of life, unveils the healing harmony - a balance of ongoing mental health enrichment interwoven adeptly with the elevating trajectory of your professional growth.

Envision a masterful musician. He doesn't just create soulful melodies; he also tunes his instrument, takes care of it, ensures it's in the best shape to produce the notes his heart desires. You, my friend, are that musician. Your life, your very existence, is the beautiful music you create. And your mind? It's your instrument. Tuning into your mental health, understanding its pitches and tonal variations, caring for your mind is as important as celebrating your professional success.

The rhythm of your work, the melody of your achievements are indeed glorious. Yet, the harmony of mental well-being you add to them makes the orchestration complete, adding a profound depth to your success saga. With each crescendo and cadence of accomplishments, if you simultaneously focus on your mind's harmonious serenade, you shall manifest an extraordinary symphony, striking the perfect proportion of professional laurels and personal wellbeing.

How does one attain this healing harmony? Well, it begins with heightening mental health literacy – recognizing not just symptomatic changes but also understanding preventive measures and therapeutic coping strategies. It stretches further to embracing validation regarding psychological help, realizing that seeking assistance is not weakness; it's wisdom. In fact, it's the sign of a proactive maestro, who wants to maintain the music of their life in perfect harmony.

Let's explore some of the ways you can bring the healing harmony to life. Embrace mindfulness as a part of your everyday routine. Whether it's seated meditation, a mindful walk in a nearby park, or merely savoring the taste of your morning coffee, be present, grounded in the moment, immersing in the sensory experiences. Such practices not only support mental well-being but also fuel your creativity, decision-making capabilities - notes that enhance your success melody.

Another instrumental strategy is nurturing healthy relationships. Maintain a steady beat of emotional connectivity with not just family and friends, but also seek out professional networks offering a safety net against work-related stressors. Foster melodic bonds that serenade a supportive tempo into your life.

Lastly, dedicate time to rest and replenish. Even a musical masterpiece needs the occasional pause - that breath of silence augmenting its captivating charm. Your life's composition too, craves these pauses. Implement a regular regimen of rest into your schedule. It's not a sign of inefficiency, instead, it's a strategic silence, breaking your work melody for a moment to enhance your mental zeal before you jump back into the rhythm.

As you climb the stairs of success, ensuring a healing harmony of mental health, akin to that refreshing interlude in an inspiring melody, fuels your journey, enriches your orchestration, and amplifies the crescendo of your accomplishments.

With the perfect rhythm of succession in harmony with a nourishing norm of mental wellbeing, you aren't just a participant in the concert of life. You are the performer, the maestro conducting a resonant rhythm of success, a melodious symphony of mental wellbeing. So, let's continue this melodious journey, as we take practical steps, and implement strategic actions to balance success and mental health.

Yes, the melody of your life doesn't just encapsulate the booming beats of success. It also reverberates the subtle notes, the healing harmony of mental health. To construct this robust rhythm, it's essential to recognize, acknowledge, and address the crescendo of challenges, tune into the healing harmony, and imbibe them into the resounding rhythm of your relentless resilience, your celebrated success.

Conducting the Concert: Implementing Strategic Actions to Balance Success and Mental Health

In the grand composition of your life, you are the masterful conductor, with the power to craft a harmonious blend of the complex melodies of success and the soothing rhythms of your mental health. As we've journeyed through the unseen struggles, the healing harmonies, it's time now to orchestrate actions that cast a magical spell of equilibrium, a concert where your success and mental well-being perform a synchronic ballet.

Understanding the symphony is the first step; the next one is to take the seat at the conductor's podium. In this part of our journey, we'll explore a few actionable methods that you can implement in your daily life to nourish your mental health while you continue to achieve great heights professionally.

First, it's about tuning your mental instrument with regular check-ups. Similar to how you get regular physical check-ups, it's equally important to evaluate your mental health. Whether through therapy, professional counseling, or self-administered mental health assessments, keeping a pulse on your mental health is vital. Regular check-ups enable you to address issues as they arise, and not when they've built up into a crescendo of overwhelming emotions.

Next, let's talk about your work's rhythm. It's easy to get lost in the cadence of deadlines, targets, and high-stakes decisions, but what's also crucial is to foster a 'success journal.' Dedicate a few moments every day to reflect on your achievements - big or small. Write them down. This practice helps you to appreciate your victories, creating a symphony of positivity and resilience.

Most importantly, it's essential to carve out mindful breaks in your day. This might mean taking a stroll in a nearby park, meditating, or spending quality time with your loved ones. These aren't distractions in your march towards success; instead, consider them as interludes, providing necessary relief and renewal for your mental health.

Implementing these strategic actions is akin to conducting the rhythm of your life's orchestra. It's about realizing that you're not just the maestro creating the mesmerizing symphony of hard-earned success, but also a nurturing caretaker of the beautiful instrument - your mind. Adding these actions to your daily routine enables you to create an effective healing harmony, where your success and mental health dance together in a rhythm of resilience, personal fulfillment, and happiness.

And remember, while implementing these strategies, always honor the rhythm of your personal symphony. We all respond differently to various therapeutic techniques and coping mechanisms. Allow yourself the freedom to experiment, explore, and settle on what suits you best.

As a high-achieving professional, you've mastered the art of taming challenges, facing high-pressure situations, and emerging victorious. Want to know a secret? That makes you the perfect candidate to ace the mental wellbeing frontier as well. With your innate courage, abilities, and resilience, you're more prepared than you might think.

Implement these strategic actions and wield the conductor's baton to orchestrate a captivating symphony that blends momentous success and enriching mental health. As we grasp what it truly means to be extraordinary performers in life, we will take these lessons forward to create a lasting encore, one that resonates with the strength of our triumphs and resilience amid challenges.

The Enchanting Encore: Embracing an Extraordinary Performer within You

In the grand concert of life, you've composed beautiful melodies of success, and you've sung the harmonious hymns of mental health. You've wielded the majestic baton, conducting the riveting rhythm of your professional victories to the soothing symphony of your mental well-being. The tunes you've tuned, the rhythms you've ridden, and the symphony you've sweetened are all echoing throughout the concert hall of your life journey. The finale has arrived, but is it really a finale? Or is it a stepping stone towards an enchanting encore?

Step back. Take a moment to allow yourself a hearty cheer for the moving masterpiece you've orchestrated so far. Let's embellish the enchanting melody of success and mental health with a resounding resonance. And that is - recognizing your extraordinary place in the concert of life.

You're not just a participant in this concert, merely tapping your feet to the tunes. You're more than a part of the audience, witnessing an array of performances. You're the performer. You're the maestro. On the grand stage of life, you're playing the instruments of success and mental health, arranging them beautifully into your life's orchestration.

Believe in this affirmation: "I am the astounding performer in the concert of life, skillfully playing the instruments of success and mental health." As this affirmation resounds within you, let it remind you that you're handcrafting a beautiful balance between professional accomplishments and mental tranquility.

Recognize and honor the unique tune that is authentically and masterfully yours. Through every high note of accomplishment and every comforting chord of mental wellbeing, affirm:

"I am not just about crescendos of success, but also the soothing melody of mental tranquility."

Celebrate your symphony for it is extraordinary.

You've embarked on a beautiful journey toward achieving the balance of professional success and mental health. Now, it's time to acknowledge the victory of orchestrating this melodic balance. As you ruminate on your concert, remember - your enchanting encore is yet to come.

The numerous melodies and harmonies are endless opportunities for growth, resilience, and happiness. The concert does not end here. It will continue, with fresher melodies, more profound harmonies, and more extraordinary performances by none other than you.

This isn't a period at the end of your concert but a comma, opening up a whole new dimension of possibilities and chapters. A moment of silencing the orchestra, only to resume with an even more mesmerizing composition. Your journey towards balancing success and mental health, while weaving an extraordinary symphony doesn't stop here. Instead, it continues to unfold into a stronger, resonating rhythm, which will reverberate powerfully into your journey ahead.

As you close the curtain for a brief moment before the riveting encore, consider this: The world awaits your performance in the concert of life. Your melody doesn't just encapsulate the booming beats of success. It also reverberates the subtle notes, the healing harmony of mental health. To construct this robust rhythm, it's essential to recognize, acknowledge, and address the crescendo of challenges, tune into the healing harmony, and imbibe them into the resonating rhythm of your relentless resilience, your celebrated success.

We've composed a beautiful symphony together. But, as all maestros know, every symphony is a step leading to a magnificent repertoire. Your next chapter awaits, a chapter where the rhythms of adaptation and resilience will add more depth to your composition, to your journey towards becoming an extraordinary performer in the concert of life. So, let's turn the page and let the rhythm of adaptability begin.

Abode of Adaptability: Breaching the Boundary of Conventional Leadership for Fostering Mental Resiliency

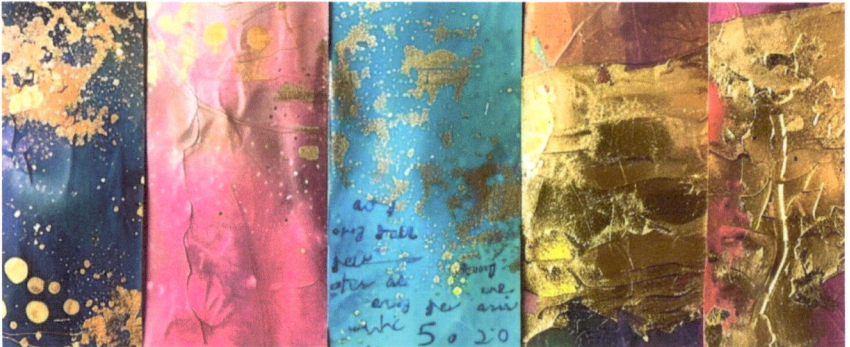

"Resilience flows from adaptability; embracing change, not as adversity, but as nature's chisel shaping us into versatile leaders of tomorrow."

Welcome, high achievers, trailblazers, and mold-breakers to a new horizon in your personal and professional journey. A place where dynamic adaptability breathes life into your indomitable spirit, where resilience flows freely from the wells of change. This chapter invites you to a transformative journey, where we venture beyond the conventional understanding of leadership, forging our path into the future shaped by mental resilience and versatile adaptation.

Navigating through the bustling cities, helming your multi-billion-dollar corporations, and leading the way in your respective fields as physicians, executives, or CEOs, you stand as paragons of success. However, beneath this triumphant façade lie your invisible battles against stress, addiction, and self-esteem issues. The relentless weight of high-pressure jobs, and soaring career demands few understand or want to acknowledge. Yet, you endure, trailblazing paths, breaking barriers, relentlessly seeking a life that's not just successful, but also deeply fulfilling and happy.

In this chapter, we are set to explore the power of adaptability. Envision adaptability not as a cumbersome pressure to conform but as nature's chisel that shapes us into resilient individuals. Like water, continually reforming around obstacles, carving its way through the hardest of rocks, adaptability empowers us with the resilience to champion our life's course. This isn't about tolerating change. Instead, it is about celebrating change, dwelling in its abode, and inviting the unfamiliar situations to weave the intricate patterns of our unique life tapestry.

You're about to embark on an odyssey where we dismantle our conventional routines, venturing into the realm of adaptability. Breaking free from the chains of comfort zones, we dare to embrace the unfamiliar, convinced in the understanding that these new experiences are the alchemy for mental resiliency. They enhance our capacity to juggle professional commitments with personal happiness, highlighting an essential premise - it's not just about surviving challenges, but thriving amidst them.

Remember, adaptability isn't a sacrifice of our core values. Instead, it's a reinforcement of them. It grants us the strength to maintain our principles amidst ever-changing circumstances, and the resilience to adapt effortlessly to life's ebb and flow. Suddenly, we are not just reactive beings but proactive pioneers. We negotiate life's challenges not as victims but as versatile leaders of tomorrow, that change is our partner, not an adversary.

"Oh, the places you'll go," said Dr. Seuss, capturing the essence of our adventure in this chapter. In the upcoming sections, you'll unravel the crucial need for adaptability, and discover the powerful interplay between adaptability and resilience. You'll understand how flexible leadership styles can impact mental health and their influence on organizational success.

This is about upgrading your life's playbook, intertwining the dynamics of success and mental well-being. Together, we'll witness the dawn of a mind molded by change, resilient in adversity, and unafraid to continuously evolve. So, are you ready to make resilience your default mode, and change your loyal companion? If so, let's embark on this exciting chapter of this transformative journey.

Venturing into the Versatile: The Inception of Transformation through Adaptability

Delving into the heart of adaptability, we navigate the intricacies of an evolving journey. High achievers, let's take a moment here, pause and reflect. Why are we even discussing adaptability? What is this noise about change, resilience, and the interplay of the two? Let's take this journey back to its roots, to unravel the compelling need for adaptability.

Consider for a moment, an oak tree. Magnificent in its grandeur, it stands, unfazed by the changing seasons. Yet, beneath its apparent stillness, it embraces change. It sheds its leaves, allowing itself to be barren during the winter, only to sprout new leaves when spring arrives. The tree doesn't shy away from these transitions; it evolves. The tree, in all its wisdom, empowers the concept of adaptability.

Now imagine, what if that tree, in its obstinacy, decided not to shed leaves in winter? Would it not drain its resources, compromising on its growth, its ability to thrive in the spring, or even survive the harsh winter?

The tree exemplifies our professional life. The ever-changing economy, dynamic corporate environments, and evolving technology - all present our professional world's changing landscapes. Stagnancy, like the tree refusing to shed its leaves, is fatal in our professional growth. Staying rooted in our comfort zones, and refusing to adapt, we drain our mental and emotional resources, preventing us from thriving amidst change.

Every change leads to opportunities– new roles, projects, or chances to advance in our careers. But they can only be seized if we're prepared to adapt, to learn, and unlearn. Adaptability, therefore, isn't just an optional trait; it's a necessary skill that caters to our professional growth. Its absence is the difference between a leader who grows and one who fails to progress despite abundant opportunities.

Now transpose the importance of adaptability to your personal life. In the chaos of navigating careers, relationships, mental health challenges, and the sweet chaos of parenthood, life is an incessant river of change. How we adapt to these changes, both significant and subtle, define the course of our personal happiness and mental resilience.

The unyielding schedules, relentless pressures, and ceaseless ambitions, have you paused, introspected, and asked yourself – are you managing change or merely surviving it?

If you're seeping in stress, finding it hard to catch a breath in your high-achievement-driven lives, maybe it's time to change the game. It's time to not just react to change after it has occurred but to anticipate it, prepare for it, embrace it, and lead it. After all, you're not just high achievers; you're game-changers. Ready, not just to lead in the professional realm, but to succeed in the personal domain of mental resilience and happiness.

Adaptability, in essence, is the antithesis of stagnation. It's the key crucial for thriving in our careers, fostering mental resilience, and achieving an equilibrium between career and personal happiness.

Ponder over this. What would our professional and personal lives be if we didn't view change as adversity, but as an opportunity? How empowered would we feel if every change, no matter how challenging, excited us, knowing it's a chance to evolve, to grow, to prosper?

That's the power of adaptability and high achievers. It flourishes our mental resilience, making us not just survivors but winners of our change-ridden odysseys. And that's the compelling need for adaptability – for its absence doesn't just thwart our growth but jeopardizes our success, our mental peace, and our personal happiness.

Let's turn the page towards understanding how this potent tool of adaptability intertwines with resilience and molds us into versatile leaders in the next section, "The Realm of Resilience: Fostering Mental Strength through Adaptability."

Abode of Adaptability: Breaching the Boundary of Conventional Leadership for Fostering Mental Resiliency

Navigating through the labyrinth of life, let's pause for a moment and reflect on the role leadership plays in the grand scheme. We aren't just talking about leading teams in corporate towers but about the leadership we demonstrate in our lives. The leadership approach we choose resonates deeply in the way we manage change and our mental well-being.

Leadership, often confined to boardrooms, is, in reality, applicable to our life's arenas. Let's unbox its real essence—an essential tool empowering us to adapt, grow, and prosper. The power not just to lead others but one's thoughts, actions, and life.

So, high achievers, let's explore unconventional leadership—adaptable leadership—the style that molds us from being managers of change to creators of it, fostering our mental resilience in the process.

Our professional life embraces change in various forms -mergers, acquisitions, leadership changes, product innovations, or shifts in business strategies. These changes can generate stress and anxiety, leading to dwindling mental peace. This is when adaptable leadership steps in, offering the resilience to navigate and lead these changes with grace and positivity.

An adaptable leader isn't just open to change but thrives on it. They see it as an opportunity to rise above the challenges, expand comfort zones, propel personal growth, and enhance team performance. By fostering an adaptable mindset, they become embodiments of resilience, reinforcing their mental strength.

Adaptable leaders operate on the mindset that "change is the only constant." They keep an open heart and mind, ready to question the status quo, learn, unlearn, and relearn. They don't just navigate change but anticipate and prepare for it, thus reducing the usual anxiety and stress associated with it. Through their agility, not just in their actions but in their thoughts, they transform change, often viewed as adversity, into a powerhouse of personal and professional growth.

Their leadership isn't about dictating their team but about fostering a culture of learning, and growth, allowing them to be resilient when faced with shifts, uncertainties, and stressors. It celebrates failures as much as successes, viewing every failure as a stepping-stone to learning, and creating a mentally healthy, stress-free work culture that fosters productivity, satisfaction, and happiness.

Taking a leaf from their book, let's transpose this adaptable leadership style to our lives. Apply the same principles while juggling high-pressure jobs, relationships, and personal challenges that life gifts us. When we become leaders of our lives, open to learning and unlearning, welcoming changes rather than fearing them, we create a life that is not just successful but fulfilling, thriving, and joyful.

So, how can we foster this adaptable leadership style and strengthen our mental resilience? Let's explore this through practical, tangible exercises to foster an adaptable mindset in the upcoming segment. But remember, the first step to growth is self-awareness—it's about knowing where we stand and where we want to be. This is our starting point, from where we embark on the empowering journey to adaptable leadership and mental resilience.

A journey where we are not just creators of our destiny, paving the way through the crossroads of change towards a life that is not just successful but fulfilling, vibrant, and mentally resilient. A journey that leads to the upcoming exploration, where we dive into the intricacies that rigid thinking patterns can bring to our lives, as we continue our odyssey through a world dominated by adaptability.

Echoes of Evolution: Understanding Adaptable Leadership

In our exploration of adaptability, we've ventured through the realms of transformation, and resilience. We've looked deeper into adaptable leadership's role in fostering our mental strength. Now, let's zoom in further and understand what shaped this evolutionary trait. It's time to unearth the echoes of evolution that have made adaptable leadership what it is today.

The dynamics of leadership, like anything else, have seen a significant shift over the years. The image of a stern boss commanding and control-ling every move has faded. What has emerged is a more empathetic, approachable, and change-friendly professional, open to diversity of thought, innovation, and employee well-being. A leader adapting to the changing times and business environment: An adaptable leader.

Undoubtedly, these leaders stand taller than their counterparts, beckoning the waves of change, not with dread, but with open arms. They are quick to alter their strategies, question assumptions, and en-courage innovation, never letting shifting climates throw them or their team off balance.

Adaptable leaders are clairvoyants, predicting change before it occurs, planning, strategizing, and proactively preparing their team for the challenges that lie ahead. This reduces the shock element when that change finally happens, minimizing the stress that usually follows. Now, that's leading change, isn't it, high achievers?

In the corporate environment, they are quick to identify shifting consumer preferences, new market trends and adjust their strategies, products, or services to cater to these changes. Rather than clinging on to once-successful strategies or decisions, they use change to their advantage. They believe in agile working, valuing constant learning, and adaptation over following set routines.

These leaders, however, do not limit their adaptability to professional endeavors. They transpose it to their personal lives as well. Being adaptable helps them navigate the ebb and flow in personal relationships, manage parenting woes, and deal with any curveball that life throws at them, ensuring not just success but happiness, fulfillment, and well-being.

As leaders who are adaptable, they plant the seed of adaptability within their teams as well. This reinforces their team's mental strength, empowering them to shift perspectives, be flexible in thinking and approaches, and remain unfazed by changes. These teams exhibit higher levels of productivity and satisfaction, paving the way for success for both themselves and the organization.

This vision of adaptable leadership certainly makes us wonder - How can we imbibe these qualities? How can we tap into this fantastic power of adaptability and become leaders of our lives? How can we create a harmonious balance between change, success, and happiness?

These questions bring us to the doorstep of our next exploration. It's time we address the elephant in the room: Rigidity. As leaders of our lives, being aware of its presence and recognizing its potential hurdles is the first leap towards mental strength. So, let's take this leap together, step onto the rocky terrains of rigidity and understand the problems it can cause on our adaptability journey. Remember, high achievers, knowledge is power, and awareness of our rigid patterns is the stepping stone to conquering them. So let's tread forward, all set to unravel the hurdles of inflexibility that lie ahead.

Ribbons of Rigidity: Unraveling the Downsides of Inflexibility

We've strolled down the memory lane of leadership evolution, pausing to wonder at the adaptability the giants of today possess. It's this very quality that makes them stand tall amongst ordinary leaders. But now, let's take a turn off this memory lane and step onto a path less traveled. Rigidity, a silent antagonist, often unspoken, are the bonds that prevent us from soaring high on the wings of adaptability.

What is it about rigidity that prevents us from progressing? Why does this mindset prove to be a challenge when change comes knocking? By looking into the crux of these questions, we are trying to unravel the downsides of inflexibility. High achievers, it's time to take off those rose-tinted glasses and confront the reality of rigidity.

A rigid individual, whether they may be running a Fortune 500 company or steering a startup, often clings to thought processes, attitudes, and behaviors that have been conditioned over time. Unresponsive to the winds of change, they choose to barricade themselves within their comfort zones instead of venturing out and exploring the unfamiliar.

This inflexibility, while it offers initial comfort, morphs into a boulder blocking the path of progress. It hinders innovation, discourages unique solutions, and cultivates a culture of complacency, hindering both personal and professional growth.

In a world that's constantly evolving, businesses led by rigid leaders risk being outdated, outsmarted, and outperformed by competitors who welcome change instead. Resistant to modify strategies that once yielded results but are no longer relevant, these companies suffer the dire consequences of stagnation.

On the personal front, rigidity doesn't fare any better. People with rigid mindsets often find themselves stuck in the rut of old habits, unwilling to adapt to the circumstances life throws at them. This leads to elevated levels of stress and anxiety, hampering mental well-being and overall happiness.

So, what do we do with these ribbons of rigidity? Do we let them tie us down, stunting our growth and potential, or do we break free, untangling ourselves towards the betterment of our lives and our mental well-being?

High achievers, as we continue our journey, our next step is to construct an agility action plan. We've confronted the reality of rigidity, now let's switch our focus towards practical solutions that we can incorporate in our lives to foster an adaptable mindset.

The power to transform rigid habits into adaptable ones is twofold. First, is awareness, acknowledging that rigidity exists, its drawbacks, and the need to change. Second, initiation, taking steps, no matter how small, towards unlearning, relearning, and learning again.

Embrace this part of the journey with a spirit of endurance as we tap into an action plan that promises a gateway to mental resilience and personal and professional growth. Let's gather the tools necessary for fostering an adaptable mindset, redefine the landscape of our lives, and imprint our footprints on the path of success with adaptability as our trusted ally.

The Agility Action Plan: Practical Steps Towards an Adaptable Mindset

We've navigated through the rigid realities of inflexibility, acknowledged its unwelcome presence, and gauged its counterproductive impacts. Now, it's time to counter this foe. After peeling away the layers of rigidity, it's time to cloak ourselves in a new skin - a skin that embodies adaptability. We've recognized the problem, now let's herald in the solution. High achievers, prepare yourselves as we pencil down an Agility Action Plan.

Lacing each step with the spirit of resilience and adaptability borrowed from our insights on leadership, let's draft this blueprint that enables us to begin the transformation at an individual level.

At first, it's about Awareness. Identify the behaviors, habits, or perspectives that are impelled by rigidity. Could it be a reluctance to delegate critical tasks, a tendency to overlook new ideas or an unwavering belief in never-changing routines? Recognize the factors in your professional and personal life where adaptability is crying out for attention.

Second, Initiate. Start with small changes, and infuse minor modifications to your daily routines. Maybe take a different route to work, change the order of your morning activities, or alter your exercise regimen. Seemingly insignificant, these modifications foster 'change adaptability', thereby conditioning your mind to larger changes in your professional or personal landscapes.

Third, welcome Diversity of Thought. Encourage different perspectives in your professional setting. The road to adaptability is strewn with diverse viewpoints and creative solutions. Promote a culture of openness and inclusiveness, where each idea, no matter how unconventional, is heard and considered.

Fourth, embrace Open-Mindedness, a crucial sibling of adaptability. Release your grip on strict beliefs, and open your mind to new possibilities, and new strategies. In personal life, it could mean experimenting with new activities, hobbies, or experiences. Professionally, it's about being receptive to innovative ideas, strategies, and processes.

Fifth, indulge in Constant Learning. Embody a learner's spirit, curious, open, and eager. Encompassing a range of subjects, from professional skills to wellness practices, learning nurtures adaptability. It fosters mental agility, making us equipped to handle changes effectively.

Finally, practice Mindfulness. Pay attention to your mental states, and emotions. Recognize when rigidity sneaks in, causing unease or stress. Acknowledging its presence is the first step to managing it. Mindfulness thus acts as a mirror, revealing when our mind sways towards the rigid end of the continuum.

As we come to the close of our Agility Action Plan, we understand there's more to leadership and success than rigidity allows us to see. It's not solely about stern commands or unchanging routines. Success, happiness, mental wellness, they all thrive in the realm of adaptability.

But before we embark on this transformative journey, it's essential to remember that this is just the blueprint. The grand design of adaptability comes to life when we step away from the drawing board and plunge into action, setting our plan into motion. As high achievers, you are in the driver's seat, steering the car of your life. It's time to reprogram your GPS, setting your destination towards the Pinnacle of Plasticity, the ultimate mark of mastering adaptability. Are you ready to turn off the highway of rigidity and cruise along the scenic route of adaptability? If so, buckle up and prepare for a rewarding ride towards the dawn of the adaptable mindset.

The Pinnacle of Plasticity: Embracing the Dawn of an Adaptable Mindset

Life is a canvas, waiting for us to splash it with our unique hues. We have examined the rigorous constraints of rigidity and the liberating potential of adaptability. We have even charted an action plan, setting the groundwork for cultivating adaptability. Now, high achievers, it is time to put our plan into action and paint our lives with the vibrant strokes of mental agility and resilience. Welcome, trailblazers, to the dawn of the adaptable mindset.

Residing at the peak of personal and professional development, the challenge of embracing adaptability transcends the mundane and elevates us to the status of pioneers. It's not just about adapting to a workplace policy or a change in living conditions, it's about evolving our very mindset, letting it flow like a river, bending and twisting according to the landscape of life. It's about striking a balance between preserving core values and adapting to the winds of change. Just like the reeds that yield to the winds yet stand upright after the storm passes, it is our ability to adapt that fuels our strength to stand, unwavering, in the face of adversity.

Let us pledge to foster an environment that breathes adaptability. From our workspaces to our homes, we can inspire those around us by embodying this dynamic trait. Guided by the affirmation, let us echo:

"I am the master of my thoughts, adapting effortlessly to life's ebb and flow. Change is my partner, not my adversary, molding me into a stronger, more resilient individual. With an adaptable mindset, I embrace every challenge as an opportunity to learn, grow, and shine brighter than ever before."

Our voyage towards adaptability, high achievers, is not marked by a finish line. It's a journey, a constant part of our lives. Each day presents a new opportunity to exercise adaptability and persistence. Each challenge is a stepping stone that strengthens our resilience and breeds mental fortitude. It's a path strewn with triumphs, defeats, lessons, and growth.

The adaptable mindset isn't aimed at eliminating stress or adversity. Instead, it equips us with the tools to navigate them efficiently. Its innate flexibility helps us transform every setback into a comeback and every quandary into a triumphant tale. It fosters a sense of resilience, boosting our mental health and propelling us further in our professional sphere.

An adaptable mindset escorts us toward a balanced life, where we are not just surviving but flourishing. It helps us pry beyond the restraints of professional success, exploring our potential for personal fulfillment. It enables us to find happiness and contentment within ourselves, allowing us to create flourishing lives that resonate with our unique essence.

After all, this journey isn't about morphing into a different person. It's about unearthing our authentic selves while acknowledging our circumstances. It's about staying true to our journey, accepting our realities, and courageously venturing into the enticing avenues of growth and adaptability.

As we close this chapter of our journey, let's reflect on what we've dismantled and what we're building. The next chapter awaiting us in our journey will navigate through the complex juxtapositions of life. As we transition into exploring how to balance our vigorous ambitions with vibrant inner peace, let's carry forward the fruits of our adaptable mindset. We've climbed the pinnacle of plasticity; now let's move ahead, tasting the sweet fruits of our labor, carrying on these lessons into our next adventure. Let's gear up, high achievers, to conquer yet another facet of our journey. It's time to weave the threads of adaptability into our fabric of life, diving deeper into the realm of inner peace, and embarking on our voyage towards nurturing vehement ambitions harmoniously.

I I

⚜

Between Juxtapositions: Balancing Vigorous Ambitions and Vibrant Inner Peace

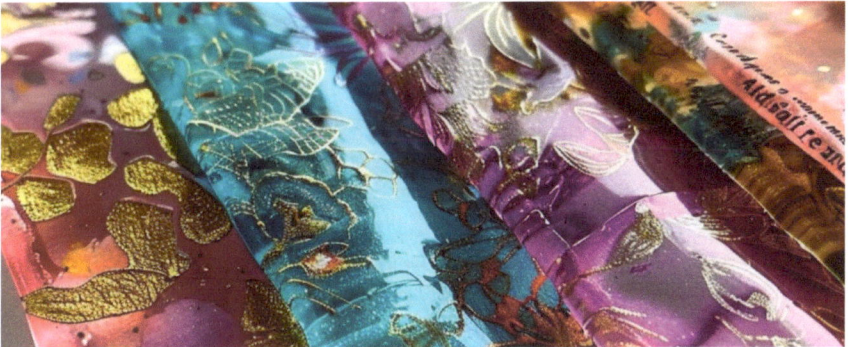

Harmoniously dance with vigor and peace; therein lies the rhythm
of fulfilled ambitions and vibrant serenity."

Welcome to a pivotal part of your journey towards balancing a high-powered, successful lifestyle while fostering a sense of vibrant inner peace. Envision yourself on a dance floor, with the rhythm of your vigorous ambitions playing in perfect cadence with the melody of your tranquil heart. Each step you take, every move you master, reflects this harmonious synchrony. What appeared at first to be a clash between two contrasting forces, vibrant peace and relentless ambition, now melodiously blend, each enhancing the magnificence of the other.

For my ambitious readers, those of you who have etched remarkable paths, heading powerful corporations, breaking ground in your respective fields as executives, physicians, or CEOs, you might perceive a complicated duality at the very heart of your success. On one side lies your desire for achievement, your relentless spirit that is forever reaching for more—more success, more accomplishment, more recognition. On the other side rests a yearning for tranquility, a vibrant inner peace that you long to nurture amidst the noise of your intense aspirations.

This chapter's guiding principle "harmoniously dance with vigor and peace; therein lies the rhythm of fulfilled ambitions and vibrant serenity," is calling for you to experience a personal revelation. It is beckoning you into a realm where your vigorous ambitions and vibrant inner peace are not polar opposites, but a harmonious twosome set on the dance floor of your life.

An ambition-fueled life does not necessitate sacrificing mental tranquility. In fact, this chapter illuminates a seemingly paradoxical truth: the more ardently you chase your dreams, the more vital it is for you to foster a wellspring of inner peace. Without this wellspring, the impressive skyscrapers of your success may stand on shaky ground. It is a delicate, intricate dance, one that calls for grace, resilience, and a profound understanding of self.

You will now begin to understand that this dance isn't intricate because it's difficult. It's intricate because it's both poignant and deeply personal. Each step you master brings you closer to a balancing point, where your professional growth and mental well-being form a beautiful dance of life, creating a rhythm that enables you to savor your success while reveling in your tranquility.

Perhaps the thought of merging these two realms, vibrant ambition and vibrant peace, seems counterintuitive. You dream of impactful achievements, yet yearn for mental peacefulness. Can these two conventions truly be in tune with each other? Allow me to guide you on a rewarding exploration that will help you answer this question for yourself. Prepare to learn this harmony dance, wherein each twirl, pirouette, or intense move, every tranquil stride or restful stillness, symbolizes the dance of your unique life.

Embark upon this enlightening journey, and you'll emerge with actionable wisdom that will fundamentally enhance the way you approach your ambitions and channel your mental peace. Consequently, you will inspire a ripple effect of positive change in those around you, inspiring them to break free from the chains of mental health struggles and to live a life of success and inner tranquility.

The promise of this chapter is simple yet profound: to help you harness the power of inner peace while actively pursuing your rigorous ambitions. It invites you to dive deep, reflect, and make conscious adjustments that harmonize your outer hustle with your inner calm. The intention is not merely to endure your life but to truly enjoy it – to thrive in the realm of achievement while cultivating sustainable serenity within your heart.

Prepare to embark on a liberating journey where the dance of ambition and inner peace forms a rhythm that guides you toward a purpose-filled life of fulfillment and tranquil bliss. As we move to our next segment, discover the distinctive canvas of your life and explore how to thoughtfully apply the palette of ambition and peace in creating your masterpiece.

The Dual Canvas: Contrasting the Colors of Ambition and Inner Peace

Feeling the pulse of a bustling city, absorbing the vibration of success and celebration, high achievers like you wake up every day to a vigorous routine steeped in dedication and relentless pursuits. It's as if you are painting on a sprawling canvas, deftly weaving the paths of your career, your dreams, and ambitions, magnifying your success with every accomplished goal. Your canvas vibrates with the intensity of dark hues —bold blues of resolve, deep reds of passion, and the midnight black of perseverance.

Paradoxically, nestled within these indomitable shades, lies a serene oasis of tranquility - a soft undertone of pastels that craves your recognition. These are the hues of inner peace— the gentle green of serenity, mild yellows of joy, and soothing lavender of tranquility. It's a solitaire realm, often overlooked amidst the frenzy of determined ambitions.

In this enthralling dance of life, the rhythmic synchrony of your poised ambition and unshakeable peace manifests itself as two contrasting colors on the canvas of your existence. One might think these contrasting elements can't co-exist, but in truth, it's their synergy that creates a breathtaking masterpiece.

This innate duality is reminiscent of Earth's day and night. The Sun and the Moon, showcasing enviable tranquility, are stark contrasts, each holding undeniable significance and adding to Earth's exquisite charm. The relentless Sun fuels life, much like your pulsating ambition fuels your success. The tranquil night invites rest—a nod to the requisite peace needed to balance the vigor of the day. It's a seamless passage, an intricate dance of two halves that whole the Earth's existence.

Our mental existence presents a similar picture: ambition is our day, peace, our night. However, lost in the routine of daytime achievements, high achievers often overlook the sacred night of peace—an untenable strategy threatening the cyclic equilibrium, shaking the stability of our mental and emotional existence.

Take a step back to appreciate your canvas - vibrant and beautiful. It doesn't just depict the high-intensity strikes of formidable ambition but also the strokes of tranquility. The merging of these contrasting colors is not just impressive but imperative, a step towards a life balanced and fulfilling, successful and joyful.

But one might wonder, how does one bring about this balance? How do we synergize relentless ambition and inner serenity? How do we paint our canvas with such an amalgamation that we create our masterpiece?

Getting there requires an understanding of the dynamics between ambition and peace, the intricate balance one needs to strike between the two. To strike this balance, we first must acknowledge both, understanding that the strength of ambition needs the calm of peace to sustain long-term.

As you journey ahead, you'll explore the nitty-gritty of this process, how to step beyond the mirage of monotony, how to become the masterful juggler harmoniously handling the spheres of ambition and inner peace. But before we venture there, take a gentle pause, delving deep into your thoughts, appreciating the sanctity of the process. This pause would ensure you are prepared to explore the thrilling circus of ambition and inner peace that awaits you in the next part of this journey. You have begun a dance, an intricate one at that, and it's essential you feel your rhythm before stepping ahead into the throbbing beats of the next segment.

Between Juxtapositions: Balancing Vigorous Ambitions and Vibrant Inner Peace

Welcome to the thrilling circus of life where you, as a high achiever, are the star performer, working to enchant the crowd with your perfect poise and balance. Your every move is a reflection of your relentless ambition, your strength, and determination. But, remember, every tightrope artist needs equilibrium, a balance between their actions and inner peace, to successfully transcend from one end to another.

Imagine your life as a tightrope suspended high above the ground, stretched between two poles: one pole representing your vigorous ambitions and the other, your vibrant inner peace. On one side, you have your formidable goals that keep you moving ahead—it's what gives your life direction and purpose. But climbing up this pole of aspirations without considering the parallel pillar of inner tranquility might lead you to a precarious fall into the mesh of stress and burnout beneath.

So, how do you maintain your steadiness on this thrilling tightrope of life? How to ensure you make it to the other end successfully, unscathed by the underlying fears of failure or imbalance? The answer lies within the poles. Much like a tightrope walker brandishing his balancing bar, you navigate through the air of ambitions tenderly, acknowledging the importance of staggering your weight equally among your ceaseless ambitions and treasured inner peace.

This approach should not be misunderstood as a mere ruthless struggle to keep the two poles at equal lengths; instead, it's your magnificent transformation into an adept acrobat who harmonizes the pulsating rhythm of ambition with the symphony of tranquil peace. It's not about pushing through the air blindly but feeling the vibes around, soaking it all in, and maintaining a rhythm that keeps you going. It's about learning to thrive, not just survive.

Remember, the sparkle in your eyes whispering the tales of your success would gradually fade if your mind is at unrest. You would nimbly leap over your towering ambitions, but the aftertaste of triumph would wane if your soul remains parched, yearning for peace. Therefore, as you glide through the tightrope of your life, ensure you anchor yourself with a robust balancing bar, beautifully adorned with sparkling ambitions at one end and a serene peaceful oasis at the other.

But bear in mind that you're not alone in this fascinating journey. Numerous artists have walked this line before you, juggling their goals while maintaining their mental tranquility, and so can you. Their victory chants should echo in your ears as you strike a balance on this tightrope, marking your triumphant journey from being relentlessly drawn towards your goals to the blissful state where you're masterfully juggling your ambitions and inner peace.

Set your sights on the far horizon, towards the pole that's gleaming with the promise of fulfillment and happiness. Take a moment as well to glance down, appreciating the depth from whence you've climbed. Know that you're not merely a performer in this grand circus called life, but the ringmaster as well. The path is yours to craft, the performance is yours to hone, and the balance is yours to find.

Are you ready to shadow the dance of other successful individuals who have walked this path and have masterfully harnessed their ambitions without neglecting their inner peace? Start preparing to be a master juggler as you ascend the pole of our next discourse, where we dwell on the art of maintaining our mental sanctity while chasing our formidable ambitions. It's about to get even more exciting in this experiential journey of life; after all, the show must go on!

The Masterful Juggler: Harnessing the Power of Ambition While Fostering Inner Calm

Imagine for a moment that you are a masterful juggler. In your hands, you have two crystal balls: one inscribed with the word 'Ambition,' the other with 'inner peace.' These elements, though seemingly paradoxical, are essential ingredients in the exhilarating recipe of successful living. The masterful juggler knows that balancing these demands indeed requires dexterity and an in-depth understanding of both forces.

Harnessing the power of ambition is like sunlight; it thrusts us into action, fuels our drive for success, and vitalizes our days. On the contrary, fostering inner calm is like moonshine; it soothes us, regulates our rhythm, and gives us tranquility amidst the chaos of our bustling day. As high achievers, we often chase the sun, forgetting that the moon, too, is a celestial powerhouse—quietly illuminating our world during our most vulnerable hours, well into the night.

Each ball you juggle exudes a distinct energy—the vigorous radiance of ambition, the soothing luminescence of inner peace. Taking turns, they rise and fall in an unending cycle, your focus shifting fluidly between each throw and catch. Sometimes we throw our ambitions higher, and sometimes we find solace in the rhythmic repetition of inner peace. It's all about the balance and rhythm.

Consider the artistry involved in juggling. Too much force, and your ambitions soar high, often too high to catch—resulting in burnout and added pressure. Too little force, and your ambitions may fall short, vibrating harshly against inner peace. To avoid such circumstances, your throw needs to be calculated and controlled; it needs to sync with the rhythm of inner peace.

For you, as a high achiever, to deal with a relentless pursuit of goals and strive for ambitious dreams, you need the tranquil nights your inner peace provides, coupling with your lunar intuition to prepare for the day ahead. Grounding yourself within this sense of calm will help you fuel your ambitions even more powerfully. Thus, fostering inner calm doesn't diminish your ambitions; instead, it offers a sanctuary, a place to strengthen your mental sentinel and emerge unscathed and more resolute.

Turning into a master juggler thus would not only shield you from burnouts but also ensure that your journey is illuminated with the promising glow of ambitions as well as the soothing light of inner tranquility. Harnessing the power of ambition while fostering inner calm is an exquisite dance, a delicate balance acquired by continuous practice, understanding, and self-awareness.

However, what if there are moments when the balls drop, and the rhythm falters? It's important to pause and reassess, for the masterful juggler isn't immune to mistakes but has the courage to pick up and begin again. When balance is lost, recalibration becomes necessary, and setbacks aren't failures—they simply offer new perspectives.

In the quest for balancing our relentless ambitions and inner peace, there also comes a moment when we need to step away from the single-minded pursuit of ambitions. The idea to recognize this moment, to transition from it, and to learn from it is what the next part of our journey explores. We are now ready to ascertain the vitality of disengaging from the relentless ambition of monotony and open the portals to enhanced mental tranquility, leading us to the path of a truly fulfilled life. Rather than swinging in extremes, find equilibrium through enlightened mindfulness that anchors us firmly between flourishing ambition and rejuvenating peace.

The Mirage of Monotony: Breaking Away from Single-Minded Pursuit of Ambition

Reflect back on the stage when you envisaged yourself as a masterful juggler, organizing the crucial facets of ambition and inner calm in simultaneous harmony. Remember the calm resilience during those slips, where the balance faltered but you courageously picked up again, recalibrating your focus. However, as with any constant practice, a vital question to ponder upon— does this single-minded pursuit of ambition and peace sometimes frolic into the throws of monotony?

In our relentless pursuit for a successful life embellished with substantial achievements and composed mental serenity, we often become engrossed in the rhythm, lost in the pattern. The single-minded mantra of continuously focusing on the goals, chasing the sun, then the moon, and again the sun, might turn into an endless loop. This constant repetition, chasing after it all, might make us immune to the beauty of our surroundings, making us oblivious to the sweet notes of life playing around us.

Picture this—you're in the midst of a captivating desert, surrounded by ceaseless sand dunes, each ridge echoing the footprints of ambitious pursuits. The sand particles reflect your aspirations, your dreams, your relentless chase towards goals. Your concentration, fixated on the crossroads of ambition and inner peace, often overlooks the oasis that might be just a few dunes away, an oasis sparkling with the opportunity to replenish and recalibrate your zest.

Sometimes in the mirage of monotony, we miss out on these oases. The path of single-minded pursuit becomes a desert wherein we overlook the intricate tapestry of life woven meticulously by webs of varied experiences. These instances offer an opportunity for pause and introspection, a chance to disengage our focus from this constant juggle.

Let's gently unclench those fists, releasing the balls of 'ambitions' and 'inner peace,' for just a moment. Stretch out your arms wide, feeling the freedom, the openness to embrace something new. This isn't a pause in your journey towards success, but an extended arm to seize more holistic experiences. A welcoming gesture to invite different strokes into your canvas. A brave step to break the mirage of monotony, an invitation to enrich your mental ecosystem.

Because, in the grand scheme of life, we aren't designed to follow a single path rigidly. Essentially, we are malleable; we are meant to sway, to experiment, to diverge from the beaten path, and chance upon off-beat trails. This sense of exploration, of embracing sporadicity of life, of absorbing a myriad of new experiences, widens our mental aperture, thereby enhancing our overall development. It is in these unplanned detours that we stumble upon the most profound lessons and experiences that truly enrich our perspective.

So, as we progress further in this journey, let's learn the art of releasing the fixation from the single-minded pursuit. Let's discover how to break away from the mirage of monotony and enhance our mental tranquility, which, in turn, elevates our sense of fulfillment. The juggle can continue, but not without giving us the joy of initiation into a more diverse and comprehensive spectrum of experiences.

With this broader perspective in mind, the journey's next leg invites you into the world of practical steps, techniques, and tools. These will guide you not only in balancing your ambition with inner peace but also in embracing a variety of experiences that pulse life into your journey. Let's step onto this exciting trail together, as we look forward to embarking on this enlightening expedition that enriches our life's tapestry, adding more colors, more stories, and more fulfillment.

The Artisan of Balance: Actionable Steps Toward Synergizing Ambition and Inner Peace

The intricate dance between our relentless ambitions and the pursuit of inner tranquility teaches us that the rhythm that guides us can, sometimes, make us susceptible to the snares of monotony. We learned about breaking away from single-minded pursuits, about crafting our unique dance— one that synergizes exuberant ambition with vibrant inner peace. But, how do we transform these insights into action, into a powerful rhythm that becomes a melody of our lives? This part of our journey provides tools on becoming the skilled artisan of balance.

Let's dive in.

Firstly, re-slotting the dials of Focus. As high achievers, our focus often revolves around our ambitions, projects, and goals. Reflect on the moments of monotonous hardships and identify the persistent trend. Likely, your focus would have been primarily persistent on the goal at hand. This type of concentration can lead to a state of imbalance. Instead, try gradually shifting your focus to include small bouts of peace-seeking activities amidst your schedule of ambitious pursuits.

Secondly, Embody Mindfulness. This involves being completely engaged in the present moment. When we obsess over our ambitions without acknowledging the rhythmic dance with serenity, we risk plummeting into a state of stress or anxiety. By incorporating mindfulness, we can learn to immerse ourselves in the present, appreciating it holistically. It is here in this present moment where we can relish the harmony of ambition and peace.

Thirdly, practice the Art of Saying No. One pitfall that goes hand-in-hand with ceaseless ambition is the inability to say no. When opportunities arise, we may feel the need to grasp them all. However, this can quickly lead to an overloaded schedule, feeding into the single-minded and monotonous pursuit of our ambitions, leaving little to no room for serenity. Learning to say no can help maintain a delicate balance, ensuring we have time for ourselves. After all, a rejuvenated mind can fuel ambitions like nothing else.

Finally, Invest in Self-Care Rituals. Incorporate practices like daily meditation, journaling, reading, or physical exercise into your routine. Disconnect from work-related stress and indulge in these practices to rejuvenate yourself. This disconnection fosters a secure sense of inner peace, giving you a fresh perspective towards your ambitions.

These are few steps towards becoming that Artisan of Balance, and indeed, there are plenty more. Remember, the goal here is to establish a rhythm, a dance between your ambitions and inner peace. In constructing this rhythm, remember to be patient with yourself, to take one step at a time, and most importantly, celebrate the small wins. Embrace the journey, relish each step, and revel in the magnificent dance of ambition and serenity.

The symphony of ambition and peace is the masterpiece that we are crafting. As we rise from being relentless achievers to becoming harmonious jugglers to skilled artisans, the impending journey promises exhilarating insights. Let's continue, ready to applaud and acknowledge our transformation, gearing up to celebrate not just our ambitions but also our victories, peace, and above all, our journey towards realizing a harmonious existence.

The Harmonious Homage: Celebrating the Symphony of Balanced Ambition and Peace

Embarking on this empowering journey, you, as high achievers and zenith chasers, transformed from relentless sprinters into skilled artisans of balance, weaving your ambitions and inner peace into a beautiful tapestry. The path teaches you to unravel the threads of experience, to tune your attention to the rhythm of balance, and to celebrate each note of the synchronized symphony of ambition and peace.

Embrace that exultant feeling that arises in orchestrated harmony, the feeling when your relentless pursuit of ambition pairs with the vibrant strokes of inner tranquility. Each victorious moment, no matter how seemingly small, holds immense significance in the balance of this dance.

Take a moment to reflect on the artisan within you, the one that crafted this intricate balance that now resonates through every corner of your life. You transformed overwhelming pressure into dynamic ambition, relentless striving into mindful pursuit, and the mirage of monotony into the undercurrent of a more fulfilling life. Every moment of self-doubt, each setback, every instance where you were on the brink of collapsing under the weight of your aspirations, you rose above it all.

Through the transformative potency of mindfulness, you learned to engage with the present moment fully, which once seemed lost in the whirlwind of your ambitions. You rediscovered the power of saying no - a tool to maintain your time and mental space and prevent them from being overburdened. You adopted self-care rituals that serve as your refuge, your oasis, in the undulating sands of your professional pursuits.

Now, it's time to celebrate this triumphant dance of life. Together, let's echo the affirmations that solidify our dedication to the harmonious future that lies ahead.

"The threads of my ambition and peace weave the colorful tapestry of my life. I am empowered, not overwhelmed. I celebrate my balanced journey— my validation lies within me, and my pace is set by me. This harmony is my strength, and my ambition, my companion, in this triumphant dance of life."

As we let this resonate within us, let's gear up for the next chapter that beckons us forward. Let's prepare to unlock the doors to an even more profound realm of inner peace against the backdrop of achievement – a kingdom of calm amidst the whirlwind of success. Taking our experiences and insights from our journey so far, we will begin transforming these accomplishments into a solid backbone, a foundation for continuing our exploration toward gaining the keys to the kingdom of calm. Anticipate a journey filled with even more enlightenment, practical wisdom, and profound experiences that will continue to amplify your personal fulfillment, success, and mental well-being. The melody of balanced ambition and inner peace continues, inviting us to dance to its rhythm, celebrating our transformation, and looking forward to the growth and enlightenment that lies ahead.

12

❧

12 Keys to the Kingdom of Calm: Cultivating Inner Peace amidst the Whirlwind of Achievement

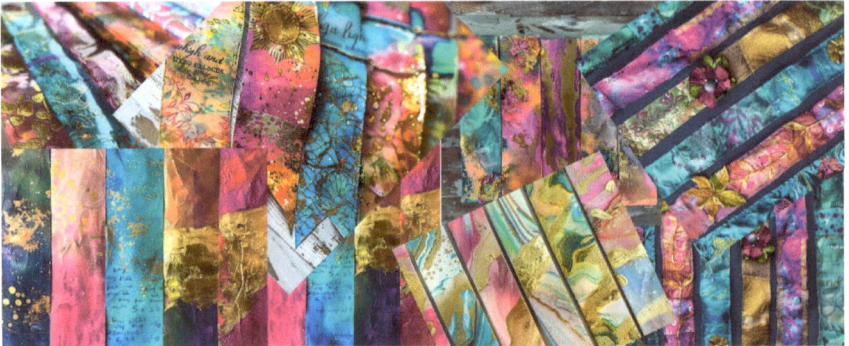

Cultivating, nurturing, and sustaining a reservoir of inner peace
amidst racing successes,
professional triumphs, and seemingly insurmountable stress.

Are you ready to embark on an audacious and transformative journey, one that doesn't lead to an elusive pot of gold but instead unlocks the door to an infinitely prosperous kingdom? This royal realm, the kingdom of calm, isn't about conquering battles; it isn't about vanquishing foes; it's about harmonizing the persistent throbs of ambition with the gentle whispers of tranquility—it's about bringing the real you to the forefront and celebrating authenticity.

In the pursuit of grand feats and astounding triumphs, high-achieving individuals know well the toll their ambitious endeavors can take on their mental health. Racing to excel professionally, maintain a perfect family life, and live up to ever-mounting expectations—they often forget to pause, to breathe, to gaze upon their kingdom from the serene hill of inner peace.

Is peace, then, a tug of war between successes and happiness—a pendulum swinging eternally between personal fulfillment and professional victories? Through this chapter, we challenge this belief. What if peace isn't a destiny but a companion, an intimate partner on the winding road to success? What if tranquility and achievement can harmoniously cohabitate, enriching your life like never before?

This chapter is your golden key, custom-fit for the heavy doors guarding your Kingdom of Calm. Here, we reveal not only why inner peace is a sturdy anchor amidst the high-pressure world of high achievers but also how you can cultivate, nurture, and sustain it—the tranquility that will accompany you in your relentless pursuit of success.

We will unravel the deepest essences of inner peace, providing you with practical insight, fun narratives, and real-world examples that take you beyond the theory and into the heart of 'living' peace. Surrounded by the roaring waves of challenges and triumphs, you will learn to remain grounded, connected to your authentic self.

Picture this kingdom—not a mythical, distant land inaccessible to many, but a peaceful abode right within you, where relentless ambition and tranquility harmoniously cohabit. The keys lie with you. You—and only you— can unlock this majestic kingdom, making it not just the backdrop of your grand story but the very essence of your being.

Are you ready to embrace a life where inner peace fuels and complements your ambitious pursuits without suffocating them? Are you ready to probe into the essence of who you really are, to cherish moments with loved ones, to break free from the chains of mental health issues, and to welcome a wave of fulfilling, purpose-driven living?

As you unwrap the first key to understanding inner peace, you'll soon realize this journey is unlike any other you've taken before. In the fast-paced, high-pressure world you navigate daily, here lies an opportunity to uncover the profound truth that success and peace are not mutually exclusive, but rather can perfectly co-exist.

In this chapter, we embark on the royal path towards unlocking the tranquil realms through the keys to the kingdom of calm. We unveil strategies, methods, and techniques to help you cultivate this much-needed serenity, enabling you to skillfully balance the whirlwinds of professional life with the gentle breezes of personal fulfillment and happiness.

Ready to embark on this extraordinary journey of self-discovery and transformation? Your royal carriage to the Kingdom of Calm awaits!

Let's begin and get ready to transition into unraveling the first key of this journey: Understanding Inner Peace.

The Mosaic of Mastery: Key 1 - Understanding Inner Peace

As a rare gem glimmers amidst the rubble, so does inner peace radiate amidst the tumultuous rush of life. Let's set sail on this illuminating journey, with the first key to your Kingdom of Calm securely in your grip—Understanding Inner Peace.

Do you recall instances when you battled an ornate dragon of stress while donning the armor of accomplishment? Or, times when waves of anxiety tried to submerge your yacht of professional triumphs? You know it all too well—you, the audacious sailor navigating the volatile seas of life. Yet, have you paused, dropped your anchor amidst the storm to appreciate the serene deep beneath the surface, the kingdom of calm, your inner peace?

Tranquility—a word often paralleled with stillness and calm, a state often glimpsed at fleeting moments of solitude or silence. But here we challenge that belief. What if tranquility isn't limited to the serene morning brew, the quiet midnight musings, or the weekend retreat to a secluded cabin? What if inner peace can thrive in your office cabin, amidst back-to-back meetings, tantalizing targets, and the constant race to the pinnacle? Surprised? Welcome to your first epiphany—inner peace is omnipresent.

Inner peace is your humble companion, walking with you, unfettered by the chaos around, consistently radiating calm amidst the tempest. It's the muted whisper urging you to pause when the world's noise becomes deafening; it's the gentle guidance pushing you to strive when the world's weight seems crushing; simply put, inner peace is the calming harmony accompanying your symphony of success.

As a high-achieving professional, understanding the essence of this harmonious companion can smooth the edges of the demanding path to success. Realizing and accepting that inner peace isn't an adversary to ambitious pursuits but a trusted ally can help balance the oft-polarizing forces of professional achievement and personal fulfillment, inspiring a life of celebratory harmony.

Peter, a brilliant surgeon based in New York, ran a race against time, armed with his surgical skills and a deep-seated desire to heal. However, amid the spiraling professional fulfilment, Peter battled invisible demons of exhaustion, stress, and self-doubt. A chance encounter with mindfulness and understanding the potential of inner peace, transformed his journey. Peter didn't abandon his ambition; instead, he invited tranquility to co-ride his professional journey. And, the harmony that ensued gifted him a life of celebratory achievements, now echoing with the silent chants of inner peace.

So, take a mindful moment, take a deep breath, look inward into the mirror of your consciousness, and acknowledge the calm radiating back at you. Your tranquil companion, inner peace, has been patiently awaiting your recognition.

As you unlock the door to the first realm of your Kingdom of Calm, allow this understanding to settle down—a professional-high can peacefully coexist with a personal calm, a racing heart can beat in harmony with a tranquil mind, and a life of bustling achievement can echo with serene whispers of peace.

Deep beneath the turbulent seas of life, lingers an eternal calm—an unshakeable, untiring, ever-present inner peace. Understanding this is the first milestone of your audacious journey—the first key to your Kingdom of Calm.

Breathe deep, soak in this understanding, and gear up as we prepare to dive deep into the Oracle of Observation: Key 2 - Developing

Self-Awareness. Get ready to unlock more secrets of lasting tranquility amidst the whirlwind of achievement.

The Oracle of Observation: Key 2 - Developing Self-Awareness

As you emerge from the calming depths of understanding inner peace, still bathed in its tranquil aura, let's dive forward into the realm of conscious existence, the Oracle of Observation. Here, we unveil the second key – Developing Self-Awareness.

In the entangled web of ambition and success, the relationship you build with your most authentic self often gets sidelined. Self-awareness, however, links this scattered ties, it's your compass in the vast ocean of personal realization, gently nudging you towards an intimate understanding of your emotions, desires, strengths, weaknesses, values, and triggers.

Imagine embarking on a dizzying rollercoaster ride, blinded. Would you enjoy the thrill, or reel under the unexpected turns? Substitute the rollercoaster with the thrilling ride of your life, the blindfold with the lack of self-awareness. Intimidating, isn't it? On this audacious journey, self-awareness acts as your sight, equipping you to face the highs and lows with informed anticipation rather than apprehensive surprise.

As high-achievers, you're akin to masterful jugglers, constantly keeping multiple balls of responsibilities, targets, and expectations in the air. While success is often measured by how well you can keep these balls from falling, wouldn't it be empowering to know which balls you genuinely want to juggle, which directly align with your authentic self and personal happiness?

Take Anika, a high-ranking executive from London. Drawn into the corporate whirlwind, Anika found herself in an intricate dance of ascending roles, plummeting personal time, skyrocketing targets, and a sinking sense of fulfillment. When she could no longer recognize the woman in the mirror, Anika turned to self-awareness. She commenced a meticulous journey of introspection, recognizing her authentic desires, strengths, weaknesses, and areas she truly wished to contribute. As Anika started aligning her professional journey with her authentic self, she started dropping the balls not contributing to her happiness. The result?: Higher satisfaction, impactful contributions, increased happiness, and a successful journey, now aligned with her true self.

On this audacious voyage, as you unveil the Oracle of Observation, let the veil of self-elusion lift. Commence the search of your authentic self, discovering what tickles your passion, what triggers your stress, where hides your strength, and how to control your reactions. Embrace every surprise, every revelation, every affirmation, and every change as you journey inwards to find the real 'you'.

Dive headfirst into this pool of insightful introspection, let the waters of determination, resilience, and enlightenment wash over you, and emerge on the shores of heightened self-awareness, your true self smiling brilliantly in the sunlight.

So take this fiery torch of self-awareness, banish the shadows of ignorance, and illuminate your journey towards the tranquil kingdom of inner peace. As you decipher the second key, remember, conquering self-awareness isn't a destination, it's a continuous journey of introspection and realization.

Have you felt the shift, the gentle yet powerful transformation seeping into your being? Embrace it, celebrate it, and gear up for the captivating journey awaiting. With this heightened self-awareness, let's tread towards a vibrant forest, the Garden of Gratitude, and learn the secrets of the Kingdom of Calm. The third key is waiting to be uncovered and promises a journey of positivity, compassion and resilient joy, enriching your pursuit of lasting inner peace amidst the whirlwind of achievement.

The Garden of Gratitude: Key 3 - Cultivating Gratefulness

Welcome! Welcome to the bountiful Garden of Gratitude! As we journey from the depths of self-awareness, we are led into the vibrant landscape of gratitude. Holding the third key in your hand, you are about to unlock the profound power of thankful reflections.

Why gratitude, you may wonder, in a journey towards inner peace? Consider this. When was the last time you savored simplicity amidst the complexity of your high-flying life? Perhaps enjoying the simple pleasure of the first morning brew, the comfort of laughter shared with loved ones, or the dazzling city lights on your way back home?

In the high octane journey of your professional life, dwelling on the oasis of these simple blessings seems almost unrealistic, even frivolous. But here, in the garden of gratitude, we challenge this thought. Let's dissect this further through the experience of Carlos, a seasoned Wall Street professional.

In the pell-mell pursuit of elusive accomplishments, Carlos lost touch with the joys of simple blessings. Consumed by stress, his vibrant spirit started to wither. His health was beginning to be compromised when he discovered the power of gratitude. He started a simple practice of acknowledging three things he was thankful for each day. This practice breathed life back into his hurried lifestyle, bringing along the forgotten joy, peace, and positive mindset. His health improved, stress lessened, and the mounting pressures of his high-pressure job were now met with renewed vigor, all nurtured by the roots of gratitude.

Gratitude, dear reader, truly is a transformative elixir. It evolves your perspective, shifts your focus from scarcity to abundance, from the unattained to the achieved, and from discontentment to fulfillment.

Reflect, acknowledge, appreciate - the simple yet powerful mantra of gratitude. Reflect on the daily blessings, however simple or grand, acknowledge their presence, and appreciate their contribution to your life. This simple practice of conscious appreciation doesn't reinvent your life; instead, it adds a vibrant tint of contentment, positivity, resilience, and, most importantly, a cultivated state of inner peace. It's like a quiet ripple that quietly transforms into a wave of positivity, infusing your life with profound peace, happiness, and zest.

So, as we unlock the third key and cultivate gratefulness remember, the garden of gratitude does not demand a colossal shift; it blossoms under the simple act of mindfulness towards one's blessings. And once cultivated it rewards you with a richer sense of contentment, positivity, resilience, inner peace and transforms your professional journey into a fulfilling personal voyage.

As we walk further on this journey of self-discovery, you, the holder of these keys, have now discovered the power of understanding inner peace, self-awareness, and gratitude. With these three keys in hand, you are better equipped to navigate the challenging yet fulfilling journey towards inner peace amidst high achievement. Now, prepare for the unveiling of the fourth secret in your quest, as we approach the mighty Fortress of Focus: Key 4 - Embracing Mindfulness. This new pursuit promises a deep dive into the present, encouraging you to focus entirely on the 'now' and the immeasurable power it holds. Stay the course, dear reader, as the secrets of the Kingdom of Calm continue to unfold.

The Fortress of Focus: Key 4 - Embracing Mindfulness

Stepping forward from the lush Garden of Gratitude, you find yourself facing the grandeur of an imposing fortress. This structure stands monumental, its massive doors tightly shut, showcasing the significance of what it conceals - your fourth key to inner peace - mindfulness, tucked away in this mighty Fortress of Focus.

Let's pause. Breathe. And think, how often do you find yourself living entirely in the present moment, unplagued by the haunting past or the uncertain future? In the race to achieve, how frequently do you pause to truly experience, understand, and appreciate the present? Rarely, isn't it?

This is the essence of mindfulness, a conscious shift of focus from what isn't to what is, from the was and will to the now. It is the practice of immersing yourself fully in the present moment, fostering a heightened awareness of your thoughts, emotions, and actions as they occur.

Consider the journey of Hannah, a renowned tech executive. Consumed by her desire for groundbreaking innovation and caught in the exhausting whirl of meetings, presentations, and decisions, Hannah felt disconnected from her present moment. With her mental well-being on the line, Hannah embraced mindfulness. She began small, taking five minutes every day to focus on her breath, on her thoughts as they floated in and out. The result was nothing short of transformational. Her stress eased, productivity and creativity peaked, and she achieved equilibrium in her high-achieving life.-

Mindfulness then is not an escape from reality. Instead, it is a conscious journey towards living in the moment. It fosters clarity, heightening your creativity, decision-making, performance, and mental tranquility amidst tumultuous pressures. Once mastered, this art of present moment awareness forms a resilient shield against stress, anchoring you firmly in the hustle and bustle of your high-achieving world.

Acquiring the fourth key, today, let's embrace mindfulness wholeheartedly. Let us strive to be active participants of our present moment, not passive spectators of a bygone past or an unforeseen future.

Dear reader, as we unlock the fourth key and soak in its wisdom, you embark on a deep exploration of the now, basking in its power and beauty. You equip yourself with a mightier tool to navigate the turbulent seas to success, knowing the power of the now is in your hands.

Feel the shift, embrace the transformation ingrained in this valuable fourth key. Rest assured, you are now four steps closer to your Kingdom of Calm, four steps nearer to harmonizing ambition with tranquility.

It's time to move forward, carrying the vibrant energy of mindfulness into the next realm of our journey. On the horizon lies a mysterious structure, concealing the knowledge of our fifth key. Keep your spirits high and your focus steadfast as we approach Stirring the Serenity Brew: Practical Steps for Cultivating Inner Peace amidst Achievement. This next part of our journey offers you a hands-on, practical approach to sustaining the harmony of ambitious pursuits with inner peace. The secrets of your Kingdom continue to unfold, and the journey continues.

Stirring the Serenity Brew: Practical Steps for Cultivating Inner Peace amidst Achievement

Moving from the fortress of focus, we journey into a mystical sanctuary that brews inner peace amidst your colossal pursuits. As you step within, you find yourself enveloped in a myriad of tools, each having the innate power to orchestrate your peace amidst your fast-paced expedition of achievements.

Inside this place, you find the sounds of serenity, whistles of wisdom, and echoes of tranquility reverberating, inviting you to sample their offerings. Shaping our fifth key, these are the practical steps to cultivating inner peace amidst achievements, the key ingredients to your serenity brew.

The first element in your serenity brew is the act of practicing meditation. Embracing meditation, akin to an ancient tree with deeply entrenched roots, allows you to remain stable and grounded in the storm of stresses and anxieties.

Remember Amelia, a seasoned lawyer? Amelia struggled with overwhelming stress, her high-stakes cases taking a toll on her mental health. Starting with just ten minutes a day dedicated to silent meditation, she wove her way towards a calmer, more centered mind, the effects of which rippled throughout her high-stakes career, allowing her to navigate the stormy seas with a newfound tranquility.

The second component of your serenity brew is positive affirmations, the language of the self to the self, instilling faith and fostering resilience. They are the gentle nudges reminding you of your capabilities, your strength, your resilience to ride the waves of high-pressure roles and responsibilities.

Next in line is the act of reconnecting with nature. This simple yet profound step assists in grounding you, reminding you of the world's rhythmic patterns and your role within them. Take your morning coffee in the garden, do your work by a window with a scenic view, or take a few minutes each day for a brisk walk in the park.

Balancing your work-life commitments follows suit. It is about optimizing your time and energy, ensuring you aren't robbed of the experiences, moments, and relationships that enrich our lives beyond professional success. It is about setting boundaries and valuing the phrase 'me-time,' cherishing small yet vital moments of self-care.

Finally, nurturing spiritual growth forms an integral part of your serenity brew. It is a personal journey that allows you to anchor on to values, principles, and beliefs that provide meaning beyond materialistic successes.

Voila! There you have it, dear reader, your own serenity brew, carefully simmered in the cauldron of wisdom, ready for you to nurture your journey towards the pinnacle of achievement while cherishing each moment of tranquility it brings.

Embrace these steps, incorporate them into your journey, and witness your serene transformation as they set you on a path towards a beautiful balance beyond professional success.

With the acquisition of this fifth key, we begin to see the full majesty of the Kingdom of Calm, a serene domain where ambitious pursuits and tranquility not only coexist but thrive. The journey, however, is just gaining momentum. On the horizon, a grand coronation awaits where you will claim your rightful place upon the throne, ruling your vibrant empire of achievement, all while gracefully cloaked in a blanket of inner peace. Hold on to your keys as the secrets of your kingdom continue to unravel, setting you on a course towards your Coronation of Calm.

The Coronation of Calm: Bestowing the Kingdom of Tranquility upon Yourself

The journey we've embarked on has taken us far. From understanding inner peace to embracing mindfulness, we've poured love, knowledge, curiosity, and boundless courage into the cauldron, and carefully brewed the perfect serenity brew.

Now as we round the bend, we make our way towards a grand stage set amidst the heart of your kingdom - the Kingdom of Calm. It's your coronation day, the moment you've been waiting for, one where you become the rightful ruler of this magnificent kingdom.

Stand tall and proud on the threshold of your Kingdom of Calm, ready to take on the mantle. As you bestow the crown upon yourself, remember the knowledge you've gained, the wisdom you've distilled, and the powerful metamorphosis you've undergone. Let the echoes of your journey reverberate between the stone walls of your majestic castle, whispering tales of strength, resilience, and the unyielding pursuit of inner peace amid a whirlwind of achievements.

Take a moment and let this sink in. Embrace your newfound wisdom; cherish the tranquility flowing in your kingdom. Now, repeat these empowering words with me:

"I am the Master of Tranquility, navigating the seas of success with inner peace as my guiding star. I celebrate this harmony, this unity of aim and serenity. The keys to my kingdom are eternally in my hand—I graciously reign over my vibrant empire of achievement, blanketed in the serene silence of inner peace."

This affirmation resonates within your kingdom walls, seeping into your heart, mind, and soul. Dear reader, in acknowledging this, you recognize your power, the strength in your resilience, and the brilliance of your tranquil spirit. You understand that your journey towards achievements can harmoniously coexist with the tranquility within your heart.

This kingdom, your personal sanctuary, exists within your reach, regardless of your external pursuits or pressures. Remember, the tools and the keys are always within your grasp, tucked away within the depths of your intellect and the chambers of your heart. Use them wisely and frequently, steadfastly nurturing your serene empire even as you reach greater heights of professional success.

As your journey continues in this Kingdom of Calm, let the tools and the keys be your loyal companions and the whispers of the wise be your guiding light. With renewed strength, clear mindset, a resilient spirit, and an armed toolkit, you are all set to navigate the turbulent seas, charting a course to unchartered territories of success, guided by the beacon of inner peace.

With the coronation ceremony complete, rejoice in the harmonious unity of ambition and tranquility. Embrace your role as the rightful ruler of your Kingdom of Calm. The journey, however, doesn't end here. A new dawn awaits, another chapter unfolds, guiding us toward redefining your perspective, redefining your journey, and fueling your continued development. As we tread this path, hold on to your crown, hold on to your inner peace, and prepare for the journey that lies ahead in our next chapter.

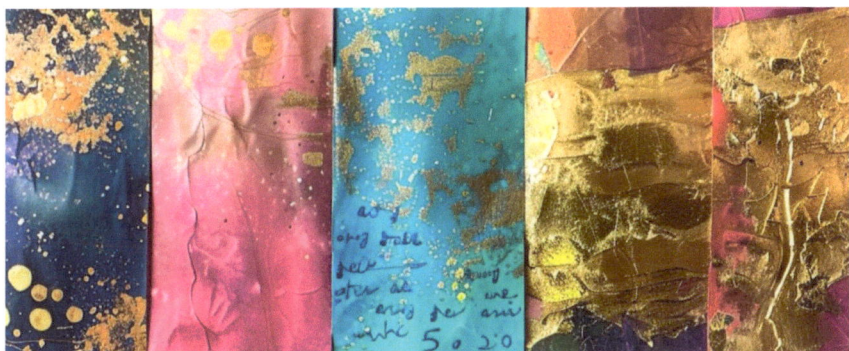

A Letter From the Author

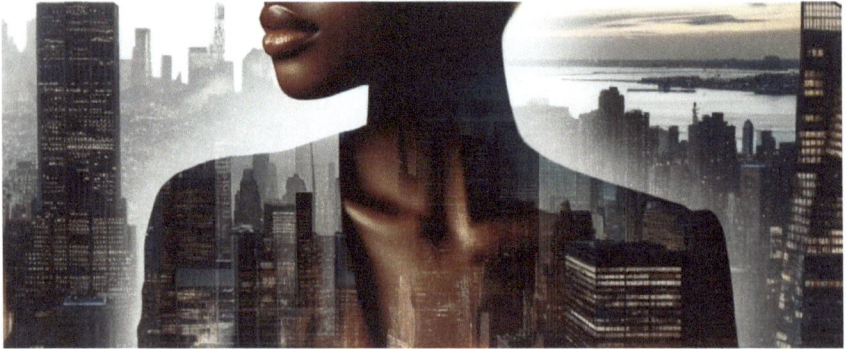

Greetings and warmest regards:

As we draw the curtains on this transformative journey through "The Mind of the Mogul," I want to extend my heartfelt gratitude for embarking on this path of discovery with me. We've ventured through the terrains of stress management, self-esteem, addiction, and the harmonization of success with serenity, each step an integral part of the mosaic that constitutes a fulfilled life.

This book was conceived as a bridge between the realms of high achievement and personal well-being, a testament to the belief that one can reach the zenith of professional success without forsaking the sanctity of inner peace. My hope is that these pages have served as a beacon, guiding you towards understanding, healing, and ultimately, thriving in a life that celebrates both your accomplishments and your essence.

Remember, the journey towards self-mastery and inner harmony is ongoing. It doesn't end with the final page of this book. Each day offers a new canvas for you to paint with your choices, actions, and reflections. I encourage you to carry forward the insights and strategies we've explored, applying them diligently to craft a life that resonates with success, peace, and fulfillment.

May the wisdom shared here ignite a spark within you to pursue a life that is not only prosperous but also profoundly satisfying and joyful. Let the lessons learned become the cornerstone of your journey, as you continue to navigate the complexities of leadership and personal growth with grace, courage, and an unwavering commitment to your wellbeing.

Thank you for allowing me to be a part of your journey. Here's to your continued success and happiness, both within and beyond the confines of your professional endeavors.

Warmest regards,
Dr. Omotola T'Sarumi

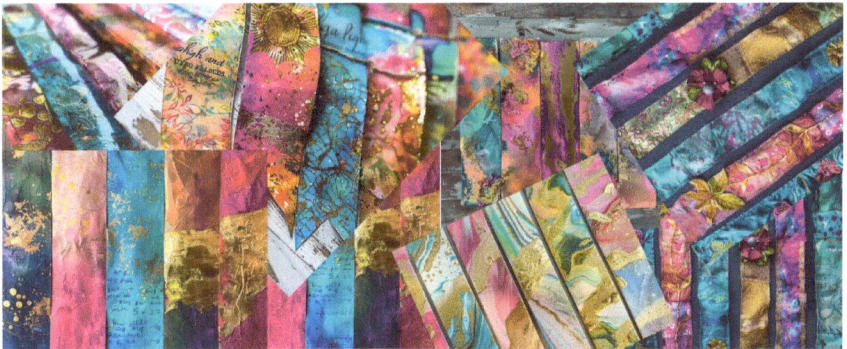

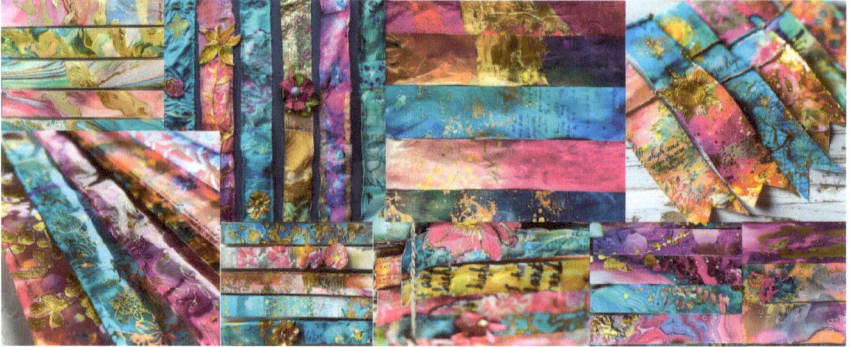

About the Author

Dr. Tola T'Sarumi is a Double-Board Certified Psychiatrist and Addiction expert who helps professionals and physicians overcome addiction, depression, and suicidal thoughts.

She's the Medical Director of Aesthetic + Mind MD, where she blends mental wellness with aesthetic treatments, offering a holistic approach to personal wellbeing. Her use of the non-invasive; non-surgical Transcranial Magnetic Stimulation (TMS) therapy has been welcomed by patients looking for a non-drug; non-shock alternative for the treatment of depression.

Dr. Tola has been tapped as an expert professional for publications, podcasts, and films, where she speaks about mental health topics, such as addiction, suicide, and depression on numerous stages. She received an award from the American Academy of Addiction Psychiatry and has also received an award from Columbia University/ NYC for her work on physician suicide, and an honoree for the Cynthia N. Kettyle Teaching Award at Harvard Medical School. She has been featured in Medscape, Forbes, the Canadian Medical Journal, the American Association of Publishing Leadership, The American Journal on Addiction, Health eCareers; The Washington Post; Authority Magazine, Thrive Global, and on podcast shows.

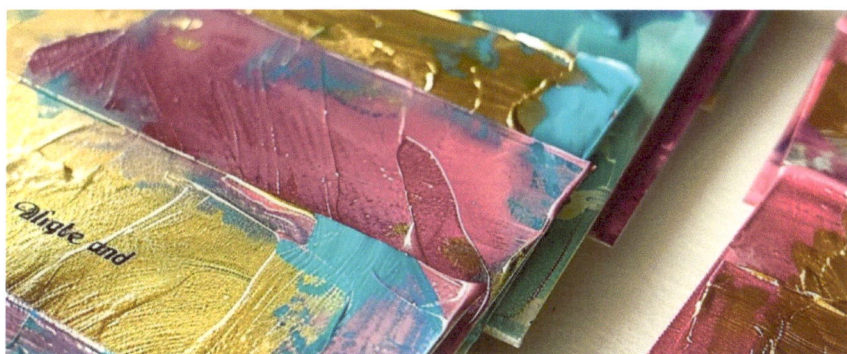

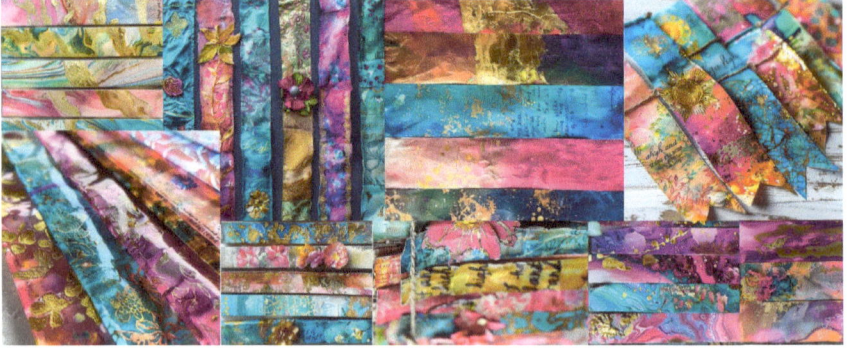

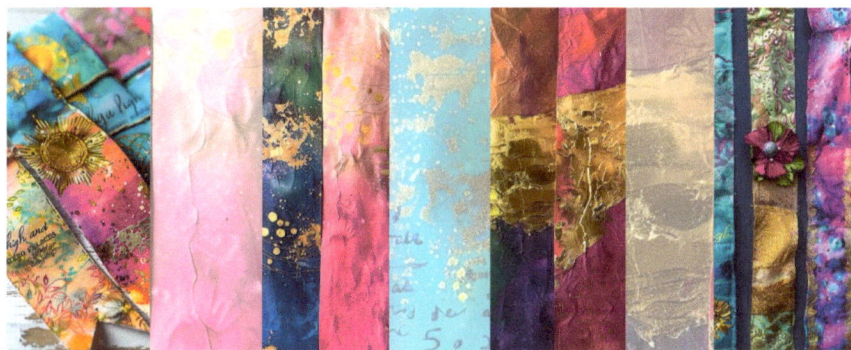

www.ingramcontent.com/pod-product-compliance
Lightning Source LLC
Chambersburg PA
CBHW041917260326
41914CB00013B/1476